Dieta cetogénica vegana

Recetas altas en grasa y bajas en carbohidratos para bajar de peso de forma saludable

Regalo gratis incluido

Como parte de nuestro compromiso de asegurarnos de que viva un estilo de vida saludable, hemos incluido un libro electrónico gratuito en el siguiente enlace. Este libro informa sobre los grupos de alimentos y los artículos alimenticios que le permitirán perder peso rápidamente. Espero que disfrute de este libro electrónico y del regalo extra también. El enlace para el regalo está abajo:

http://36potentfoodstoloseweightandlivehealthy.gr8.com

Descargo de responsabilidad

TABLA DE CONTENIDO

5

6

Sobre el autor

Sam Kuma es un apasionado de compartir su experiencia culinaria con el mundo. Su trabajo implica la modernización de los planes de dieta saludable. Ha publicado muchos libros de recetas de cocina vegana, cetogénica, paleo-dietética y de comida rápida, junto con varios libros de cocina sobre cocinas étnicas. Su enfoque principal es hacer que las dietas saludables como la vegana y la cetogénica sean la corriente principal, compartiendo recetas fáciles de crear y apetitosas. En sus dos primeros libros sobre recetas veganas, ha producido deliciosos chocolates, postres, helados, hamburguesas y sándwiches veganos.

Descripción del libro

La dieta cetogénica es una dieta basada en grasas que tiene como objetivo controlar la ingesta de carbohidratos. Es una dieta de pérdida de peso que está diseñada para ayudar a las personas a perder el exceso de peso. Este libro ha sido escrito para satisfacer las necesidades de aquellos que se suscriben a la dieta vegana y por lo tanto proporciona recetas cetogénicas veganas simples.

El libro también proporciona un plan de comida cetogénica de 15 días que le permitirá iniciar su dieta. Estoy seguro de que hay muchos libros por ahí basados en la dieta Cetogénica, pero ninguno de ellos es tan completo e informativo como este.

El libro es fácil de navegar y ha sido escrito para una lectura conveniente. Estas son algunas de las características del libro

- Recetas simples que pueden ser preparadas por casi cualquier persona.
- Recetas que usan ingredientes simples que son fácilmente disponibles.
- Un delicioso menú de desayuno.
- Un menú de almuerzo y cena diseñado para satisfacer un amplio paladar.
- Recetas simples de desayuno.

- Un completo plan de comidas de 15 días para empezar.

Una vez que usted comience con la dieta, comenzará a experimentar una variedad de cambios tanto dentro como fuera de su cuerpo. Este libro tiene como objetivo ayudarle a experimentar esos cambios y guiarle a través de una transformación permanente.

Entonces, ¿qué está esperando? Empiece con este libro hoy.

Introducción

En primer lugar, le agradezco que haya elegido este libro y espero que se divierta leyéndolo. La salud es uno de los aspectos más importantes de la vida. Si da su salud por sentada, entonces está obligado a sufrir las consecuencias. Por lo tanto, es importante centrarse en la buena salud y eliminar el estrés innecesario.

Una buena manera de hacerlo es siguiendo una dieta estricta. Una dieta puede ayudarlo a perder peso y a mantener un cuerpo ideal. Cuando escuchamos la palabra "dieta" la mayoría de nosotros asumimos que debemos lidiar con alimentos suaves como sopas y guisos. Sin embargo, no todas las dietas requieren que usted se conforme con este tipo de alimentos; una de ellas es la dieta cetogénica. La dieta Cetogénica fue diseñada originalmente para ayudar a los pacientes de epilepsia a controlar sus ataques, pero pronto los médicos comenzaron a identificar su impacto positivo en la pérdida de peso. Empezaron a administrar la dieta a pacientes obesos y notaron que experimentaban resultados positivos con ella. Desde entonces, la dieta ha sido ampliamente utilizada como una dieta de pérdida de peso.

La dieta cetogénica promueve el consumo de grasas que son buenas para el cuerpo mientras reduce el consumo de carbohidratos. Los carbohidratos son requeridos por el cuerpo para llevar a cabo las actividades diarias. Sin embargo, una dieta moderna es tan alta en carbohidratos que no se agotan en un día. El repuesto se almacena en el cuerpo en forma de grasa. Esta grasa a veces puede convertirse en grasa visceral, que es difícil de aflojar y eliminar. El resultado será un cuerpo obeso que es incapaz de quemar los depósitos excesivos de grasa.

La dieta Cetogénica tiene como objetivo eliminar tal situación. Ayuda a reducir los carbohidratos que se convierten en grasa y promueve el consumo de grasa buena que ayuda a descomponer la grasa almacenada. Existe un concepto erróneo generalizado de que la dieta cetogénica está basada en la carne. Sin embargo, se puede modificar para adaptarse a los gustos tanto de los vegetarianos como de los veganos.

La dieta cetogénica vegana promueve el consumo de frutas frescas, vegetales y granos enteros que no han sido procesados químicamente. Prohíbe estrictamente el consumo de comida chatarra y alimentos procesados que son capaces de llenar el cuerpo con toxinas. Aparte de la pérdida de peso, la dieta cetogénica proporciona una gran cantidad de otros beneficios que son grandes para el cuerpo. Algunos de estos incluyen la lucha contra enfermedades como el cáncer y las enfermedades cardiovasculares, mejorar la salud de la piel y el cabello, aumentar la energía y construir una fuerte inmunidad.

La dieta es bastante simple de adoptar y cualquiera puede tomarla. No es necesario introducir un mundo de cambios en su dieta actual para adoptar la dieta Cetogénica. Solo hay que hacer pequeños cambios para incorporarlo.

Comience analizando su dieta actual e identificando la cantidad de carbohidratos que está ingiriendo. A continuación, calcule exactamente cuánto necesita en el día a día. Elabore un plan de ejercicios que le ayude a perder el exceso de libras mientras quema los carbohidratos consumidos.

Para que empiece a conocer las comidas que debe consumir en la dieta, este libro proporciona recetas cetogénicas sencillas que le darán una ventaja y le llevarán por el buen camino. Han sido probados y diseñados para adaptarse a un amplio paladar. También proporciona un plan de comidas de 15 días que ha sido diseñado para satisfacer las necesidades de aquellos que desean perder el exceso de peso en poco tiempo.

Espero que utilice este libro para experimentar resultados positivos y cambiar la forma en que se ve y se siente sobre usted mismo.

¡Comencemos!

Plan de comidas de 15 días

Día 1

Desayuno - Panqueques de proteína Keto

Almuerzo - Sopa de crema de brócoli

Merienda - Keto Hummus

Cena - Pan Vegano

Postres - Keto Fudge super fácil

Día 2

Desayuno - Cereal de desayuno Keto

Almuerzo - Sopa ligera de calabacín

Snack - Palomitas de Coliflor

Cena - Risotto de calabaza y queso cheddar bajo en carbohidratos

Postres - Pudín de chocolate

Día 3

Desayuno - Bol de desayuno

Almuerzo - Ensalada griega

Merienda – Papas fritas de chirivía

Cena - Tofu con salsa tailandesa de coco y maní

Postres - Mousse de fresa

Día 4

Desayuno - Leche de Coco Cremosa con Bayas

Almuerzo - Ensalada de Tempeh

Snack - "Cuñas de patata" de búfalo

Cena - Pad Thai baja en carbohidratos

Postres - Galletas de azúcar Veganas Keto

Día 5

Desayuno – Barras de desayuno con tarta de queso

Almuerzo - Boloñesa picante de champiñones y nueces

Snack - Barras de granola

Cena - Ensalada de Atún Simulada

Postres - Muffins de pan de jengibre con cetona vegana

Día 6

Desayuno - Revuelto de Tofu

Almuerzo - Rollos de calabacín con coliflor y puré de brócoli

Snack - Almendras picantes

Cena - Ensalada de col morada y nuez

Postres – Rebanada de dulce de leche y chocolate sin hornear

Día 7

Desayuno - Panqueques indios salados

Almuerzo - Lasaña de berenjena

Snack - Papas fritas de berenjena

Cena - Sopa de zanahoria y calabacín

17

Postres - Mini Tarta de Calabaza con Mantequilla de Cacahuete de bajo contenido en carbohidratos

Día 8

Desayuno - Taza de café y coco

Almuerzo - Sopa cremosa de tomate sin crema

Snack - Papas fritas de calabacín ahumado

Cena - Arroz con Coliflor Mexicano

Postres - Pudín de Chocolate Chia

Día 9

Desayuno – Chocolate caliente que acelera el metabolismo

Almuerzo - Bol de Taco de Jaca y Coliflor

Snack - Wraps de Lechuga

Cena - Sopa agridulce china

Postres - Brownies Veganos de Proteína Keto

Día 10

Desayuno - Batido verde

Almuerzo - Tofu crujiente prensado con ajo y menta

Snack - "Cuñas de patata" de búfalo

Cena - Tofu de almendras picantes

Postres - Bolas de proteína de arándanos con nuez

Día 11

Desayuno - Batido de proteínas de cereza y chocolate

Almuerzo – Wraps de col rizada

Snack - Palomitas de Coliflor

Cena - Bol de fideos con curry cremoso

Postres – Helado vegano de Mantequilla de maní con chocolate bajo en carbohidratos

Día 12

Desayuno - Batido de vainilla

Almuerzo - Shiritaki "Alfredo" con espinacas

Snack - Edamame de soja y sésamo

Cena - Moussaka vegano

Postres - Paletas de fresa y limón

Día 13

Desayuno - Batido de la Diosa Verde

Almuerzo - Wraps de Lechuga Tempeh

Snack - Barcos de ensalada de amapola de limón y Tahini

Cena - Sopa de crema de champiñones

Postres - Galletas de azúcar Veganas Keto

Día 14

Desayuno - Batido de frutas

Almuerzo - Sopa de coliflor

Merienda - Keto Hummus

Cena – Masa de pizza vegetariana

Postres - Pudín de chocolate

Día 15

Desayuno - Batido de melón

Almuerzo - Vegan Keto Lo Mein

Snack - Barras de granola

Cena - Cigkofte Vegano

Postres - Muffins de pan de jengibre con cetona vegana

Capítulo 1: Recetas cetogénicas de desayuno vegano

Panqueques de proteína Keto

Preparación: 10 min	Total: 30 min	Porciones: 8-12

Ingredientes:

- 2 cucharadas de polvo de proteína vegetal
- 4 cucharadas de polvo de cáscara de psyllium, remojado en una taza de agua
- 2 cucharadas de aceite de coco
- 2 cucharaditas de polvo de hornear
- ½ taza de harina de coco
- 2 tazas de agua
- 2 cucharaditas de extracto de vainilla

Instrucciones:

1. Añada aceite de vainilla y coco a la cáscara de psyllium, que está empapada en agua. Mezcle bien y déjelo reposar un tiempo.
2. Mezcle en un tazón grande, proteína en polvo, polvo de hornear y harina de coco.
3. Añada agua y mezcle bien.

4. Añada la mezcla de psyllium en el tazón y mezcle hasta que esté bien combinado.
5. Coloque una sartén antiadherente a fuego medio. Vierta sobre ¼ de taza de masa sobre la sartén. Agite la sartén para que la masa se extienda un poco.
6. Cocine hasta que la parte inferior esté dorada. Voltee los lados y cocine el otro lado también.
7. Repita los dos pasos anteriores con la masa restante.

Cereales Keto para el desayuno

Preparación: 15 min	Total: 17 min	Porciones: 2

Ingredientes:

- ¼ taza de nueces, picadas
- ¼ taza de nueces, picadas
- 1/3 tazas de almendras, picadas
- ¼ taza de arándanos
- 4 fresas, picadas
- Edulcorante (Stevia o Splenda) al gusto (opcional)
- Leche de coco o leche de almendras para servir

Instrucciones:

1. Mezcle todos los ingredientes en un bol. Dividir en 2 tazones y servir con leche de almendras o leche de coco.

Bol de desayuno

Preparación: 10 min	Total: 12 min	Porciones: 4

Ingredientes:

- 2 aguacates medianos, pelados, sin semilla, partidos por la mitad
- 4 cucharadas de tahín
- 1 zanahoria grande, rallada

Para el aliño:

- 2 cucharadas de jugo de limón
- 2 cucharadas de aceite de oliva virgen extra
- ½ cucharadita de jengibre rallado
- ½ cucharada de semillas de amapola
- 1/8 de cucharadita de sal

Instrucciones:

1. Bata todos los ingredientes del aderezo en un recipiente. Deje la mezcla a un lado por un tiempo para que los sabores se fijen.

2. Tome ¼ de taza del aderezo y añádalo en un tazón. Añada las zanahorias. Mezcle bien. Puede usar el resto del aderezo en una ensalada.
3. Rellene las mitades de aguacate con él.
4. Cubrir con Tahini y sirva.
5. Cúbralo con la otra mitad del aguacate y disfrute.

Leche de Coco Cremosa con Bayas

Preparación: 2 min	Total: 3 min	Porciones: 1

Ingredientes:

- ½ taza de frutos del bosque (moras, frambuesas o fresas) frescas o congeladas
- 2 onzas de almendras
- 1 taza de crema de leche de coco
- 1 pizca grande de canela

Instrucciones:

1. Mezcle todos los ingredientes en un bol.
2. Sirva. Se recomienda servirlo frio.

Barras de Desayuno con Tarta de Queso

Preparación: 5 min	Total: 30 min	Porciones: 4

Ingredientes:

- 2 onzas de queso crema vegano, suavizado
- ¼ de taza de leche de coco en lata
- 1 cucharada de polvo de proteína de guisante de vainilla
- ½ cucharadita de canela molida para espolvorear
- 1 cucharada de mantequilla vegana, suavizada
- 2 cucharadas de Swerve o cualquier otro edulcorante granulado
- 1 cucharada de harina de coco

Instrucciones:

1. Añada el queso crema, la mantequilla y mézclelo en un recipiente. Bata hasta que esté cremoso.
2. Agregue la leche de coco y mezcle bien. Añada la harina de coco y la proteína en polvo; y vuelva a mezclar.
3. Transfiera toda la mezcla a una pequeña bandeja para hornear engrasada. Espolvoree canela por encima.

4. Hornee en un horno precalentado a 350° F durante unos 20 minutos o hasta que esté listo.
5. Corte y sirva.

Revuelto de Tofu

Preparación: 20 min	Total: 30 min	Porciones: 2-3

Ingredientes:

- 16 onzas de tofu extra firme
- 1 cebolla roja, en rodajas finas
- 1 pimiento rojo mediano, finamente picado
- 4 tazas de col rizada, retire los tallos duros y las costillas, picadas en trozos grandes
- 1 cucharadita de comino en polvo
- 2 cucharadas de aceite de oliva
- ½ cucharadita de polvo de cúrcuma
- 1 cucharadita de ajo en polvo
- ½ cucharadita de chile en polvo
- 1 cucharadita de sal marina o al gusto
- 1 cucharada de cilantro fresco picado
- Salsa baja en carbohidratos para servir (opcional)
- Un toque de salsa picante

Instrucciones:

1. Coloque el tofu sobre capas de papel toalla. Coloque una bandeja de fondo grueso sobre ella para que el exceso de humedad sea absorbido por

el papel toalla. Deje que se quede en esta posición durante unos 15 o 20 minutos.

2. Cuando esté listo, retire la olla y desmenuce el tofu en trozos del tamaño de un bocado.

3. Mezcle en un bol pequeño todas las especias secas y 2 o 3 cucharadas de agua y déjelas a un lado.

4. Coloque una sartén a fuego medio. Añada el aceite y caliéntelo. Añada las cebollas y el pimiento rojo y cocine hasta que las cebollas estén translúcidas.

5. Añada la col rizada, la sal y la pimienta. Mezcle bien, cubra y cocine por unos 2 minutos.

6. Coloque las verduras a un lado de la sartén y añada el tofu. Saltee el tofu durante un par de minutos y vierta la mezcla de especias sobre el tofu y las verduras. Luego, mezcle el tofu y las verduras hasta que estén bien combinadas.

7. Cocine durante 6-7 minutos.

8. Añada la salsa picante y mezcle.

9. Adorne con cilantro y sirva.

Panqueques indios salados

Preparación: 15 min	Total: 35 min	Porciones: 8

Ingredientes:

- 2 tazas de leche de coco con toda la grasa
- 1 taza de harina de tapioca
- 1 taza de harina de almendra
- 1 cebolla roja, picada
- 2 pimientos serranos, picados
- ½ cucharadita de polvo de cúrcuma
- ½ cucharadita de chile Kashmiri en polvo
- 1 ½ cucharaditas de sal o al gusto
- Trozos de 1 pulgada de jengibre, pelados, rallados
- ¼ taza de hojas de cilantro fresco
- Pimienta en polvo a gusto
- Aceite de coco o ghee o aceite de oliva para hacer panqueques

Instrucciones:

1. Agregue la harina de almendra, la harina de tapioca, la cúrcuma en polvo, la sal, la pimienta en polvo y el chile Cachemira en polvo en un recipiente.

2. Mezcle bien y añada la leche de coco. Bátalo hasta que esté bien combinado.
3. Añada la cebolla, el cilantro, el chile serrano y el jengibre.
4. Coloque una sartén antiadherente a fuego medio. Añada una cucharadita de aceite de ½. Vierta alrededor de un cucharón lleno de masa en la sartén. Agite la sartén para extender la masa. Cocine hasta que la parte inferior esté dorada. Voltee los lados y cocine el otro lado también.
5. Haga panqueques con la masa restante siguiendo el paso 4.

6. Sirva con menta o chutney de cilantro.

Taza de café y coco

Preparación: 5 min	Total: 7 min	Porciones: 1

Ingredientes:

- ¼ taza de linaza molida,
- ¼ taza de copos de coco, sin azúcar
- 2 cucharadas de aceite de coco
- 1 taza de café negro caliente, sin azúcar
- Edulcorante líquido al gusto

Instrucciones:

1. Añada todos los ingredientes en un bol. Bátalo hasta que esté bien combinado.

2. Vierta en una taza y sirva.

Chocolate caliente que acelera el metabolismo

Preparación: 3 min	Total: 10 min	Porciones: 2

Ingredientes:

- 2 cucharadas de proteína de chocolate vegetariana en polvo
- ½ cucharadita de canela molida
- Una pizca de pimienta en polvo
- ¼ de taza de leche de coco en lata
- ¼ cucharadita de pimienta de cayena, picada
- 2 tazas de agua

Instrucciones:

1. Vierta el agua en una olla y caliéntela hasta que casi hierva. Retire la olla del fuego.
2. Divida la leche de coco y las especias en 2 tazas. Vierta un poco de agua en la taza y mezcle bien.
3. Divida y agregue el polvo de chocolate y vierta el agua restante. Mezcle bien y sirva.

Batido Verde

Preparación: 8 min	Total: 10 min	Porciones: 2

Ingredientes:

- 4 tazas de espinacas
- 2 tazas de leche de coco, refrigerada, sin azúcar
- 4 nueces de Brasil
- 2/3 taza de almendras
- 2 cucharadas de cáscara de psyllium
- 2 cucharadas de polvo de proteína vegetal
- 2 cucharadas de polvo verde
- 4 gotas de Stevia o al gusto (opcional) o cualquier otro edulcorante de su elección

Instrucciones:

1. Añada las espinacas, las almendras, las nueces de Brasil y la leche de coco a la licuadora y licúe hasta que esté suave.
2. Añada el resto de los ingredientes y mezcle hasta que esté suave y cremoso.
3. Viértalo en vasos altos.
4. Sirva inmediatamente con hielo picado.

Batido de proteína de cereza y chocolate

Preparación: 8 min	Total: 10 min	Porciones: 2

Ingredientes

- 2 tazas de leche de coco, sin azúcar
- ¼ taza de cerezas frescas, sin semilla (Si usa congeladas, descongélelas)
- 2/3 taza de corazones de cáñamo
- 2 cucharadas de polvo de proteína vegetal
- ½ taza de cacao en polvo, sin azúcar
- 1 cucharadita de Stevia de chocolate líquido o al gusto

Instrucciones:

1. Añada todos los ingredientes a la licuadora y bata hasta que esté suave.
2. Viértalo en vasos altos y sírvalo con hielo picado.

Batido de vainilla

Preparación: 5 min	Total: 7 min	Porciones: 1

Ingredientes:

- 1 cucharada de semillas de chía o 1 cucharada de mantequilla de coco
- ½ taza de leche de coco
- 2 cucharadas de polvo de proteína vegetal
- ½ cucharada de aceite de coco extra virgen
- ½ cucharadita de extracto de vainilla
- 3-4 gotas de Stevia o al gusto
- 3 cucharadas de agua

Instrucciones:

1. Añada todos los ingredientes en una licuadora y mezcle hasta que esté suave.
2. Viértalo en un vaso. Sirva con hielo picado inmediatamente.

Batido de la Diosa Verde

Preparación: 10 min	Total: 12 min	Porciones: 2

Ingredientes:

- 1 aguacate, pelado, sin hueso, picado
- 1 ¼ tazas de leche de coco
- ½ taza de espinacas frescas, enjuagadas
- ½ taza de hojas de menta fresca, enjuagadas
- 2 cucharadas de polvo de proteína de vainilla vegana (o natural)
- ¼ taza de pistachos, sin sal
- 2 cucharaditas de extracto de vainilla
- 6 -10 gotas de Stevia líquida
- 1 taza de agua de coco o agua corriente
- Pocos cubitos de hielo

Instrucciones:

1 Añada todos los ingredientes en una licuadora. Mezcle hasta que esté suave y cremoso.
2 Transfiera el batido a vasos altos.
3 Añada hielo picado y sirva.

Bol de batido de Matcha

Preparación: 5 min	Total: 7 min	Raciones: 2

Ingredientes:

- 3 cucharadas de bayas de goji
- 2 cucharaditas de polvo de Matcha
- 2 cucharadas de plumillas de cacao
- 3 cucharadas de semillas de chía
- 2 cucharadas de copos de coco
- 2 tazas de yogur de coco
- 2 cucharadas de polvo de verduras (opcional)

Instrucciones:

1. Añada el polvo de Matcha, el polvo de verduras si lo usa y el yogur en una licuadora y bata hasta que esté suave.
2. Viértalo en 2 bol. Añada semillas de cacao, semillas de chía y las hojuelas de coco.
3. Mezcle, deje enfriar un poco y sirva.

Batido de bayas

Preparación: 5 min	Total: 7 min	Porciones: 2

Ingredientes:

- 1 ¼ tazas de leche de coco, sin azúcar
- 1 ½ tazas de leche de almendras, sin azúcar
- ½ taza de arándanos, frescos o congelados
- ½ taza de frambuesas, frescas o congeladas
- ½ taza de fresas, frescas o congeladas
- ½ taza de nueces
- Hielo según sea necesario

Instrucciones:

1 Añada fresas, arándanos, frambuesas, nueces, leche de coco y leche de almendras a la licuadora.
2 Mezcle hasta que el batido esté suave y cremoso.
3 Transfiera el batido a dos vasos altos.
4 Añada hielo picado y sirva.

Batido de melón

Preparación: 8 min	Total: 10 min	Porciones: 1

Ingredientes:

- 1 taza de trozos de melón
- ½ taza de fresas, picadas
- 4-5 hojas de lechuga romana

Instrucciones:

1. Añada todos los ingredientes a la licuadora y licue hasta que esté suave. Añada más agua para diluir el batido si desea un batido de consistencia más ligera.
2. Viértalo en vasos altos.
3. Sirva con hielo picado.

Batido saludable para el corazón

Preparación: 10 min	Total: 12 min	Porciones: 3

Ingredientes:

- 2 tazas de col roja picada
- 2 tomates roma
- 10 fresas medianas, picadas
- 1 pimiento rojo, picado
- 1 taza de frambuesas
- 2 tazas de agua fría

Instrucciones:

1 Añada todos los ingredientes a una licuadora y bata hasta que esté suave. Agregue más agua para diluir el batido si desea un batido de consistencia más ligera.
2 Vierta en vasos altos.
3 Sirva con hielo.

Capítulo 2: Recetas de sopa vegana cetogénica

Sopa de crema de brócoli

Preparación: 15 min	Total: 30 min	Porciones: 6

Ingredientes:

- 1 coliflor grande, cortada en pedazos
- 6 tazas de brócoli, finamente picado
- 2 cebollas amarillas en rodajas
- 2 cucharaditas de aceite de oliva virgen extra
- 5 tazas de leche de almendras, sin azúcar
- 1 ½ cucharaditas de sal marina
- Pimienta negra recién molida
- 2 cucharadas de cebolla en polvo

Instrucciones:

1. Coloque una olla grande a fuego medio. Añada aceite. Cuando el aceite se caliente, añada las cebollas y saltéelas hasta que las cebollas estén translúcidas. Añada sal, pimienta, coliflor y leche. Mezcle y deje que hierva.

2. Baje la temperatura y cubra con una tapa. Cocine a fuego lento hasta que esté suave. Añada la mitad del brócoli y retírelo del fuego. Déjelo reposar por un tiempo.
3. Transfiéralo a una licuadora y mezcle hasta que esté suave. Transfiéralo nuevamente a la olla.
4. Añada el brócoli y la cebolla en polvo restantes y revuelva. Ponga la olla de nuevo en el fuego y cocine a fuego lento hasta que el brócoli esté tierno.
5. Sirva en tazones de sopa. Sirva caliente.

Sopa ligera de calabacín

Preparación: 5 min	Total: 20 min	Porciones: 2

Ingredientes:

- 1 calabacín mediano, cortado en cubos
- 2 tazas de caldo vegetal
- 1 cebolla pequeña, picada
- 1 pimiento pequeño, picado
- Sal al gusto
- Pimienta
- ¼ taza de eneldo fresco, picado
- 1 cucharada de aceite de oliva

Instrucciones:

1. Coloque una olla a fuego medio. Añada aceite. Cuando se caliente el aceite, añada las cebollas y la pimienta. Saltee hasta que las cebollas estén translúcidas.
2. Añada el caldo, la sal y la pimienta. Cocine a fuego lento durante 8-10 minutos. Añada el calabacín y cocine a fuego lento hasta que esté tierno. Retírelo del calor.
3. Añada eneldo y sirva caliente o frío. Si desea servirlo frio, colóquelo en la nevera.

Sopa fría de aguacate

Preparación: 10 min	Total: 12 min	Porciones: 4-5

Ingredientes:

- 3 tazas de puré de aguacate Hass
- 3 tazas de caldo de verduras
- 1 taza de crema de coco (opcional)
- ½ taza de cilantro, picado
- 2 pimientos jalapeños, sin semillas, picados
- 2 cucharaditas de comino molido
- 1 cucharadita de sal o al gusto

Instrucciones:

1. Añada todos los ingredientes a la licuadora y licue hasta que esté suave.
2. Deje enfriar hasta su uso.
3. Sirva en tazones individuales.

Sopa de crema de champiñones

Preparación: 10 min	Total: 40 min	Porciones: 2

Ingredientes:

- 3 tazas de coliflor, cortada en pedazos.
- 2 tazas de leche de almendras sin azúcar
- 1 ½ cucharaditas de polvo de cebolla
- ½ cucharadita de sal de roca del Himalaya
- Pimienta recién molida, a gusto
- 1 cucharadita de aceite de oliva extra virgen
- 2 ½ tazas de champiñones blancos, en rodajas
- 1 cebolla amarilla picada
- ½ cucharadita de ajo en polvo

Instrucciones:

1 Coloque una olla a fuego medio. Añada el ajo, la coliflor, la leche, la cebolla en polvo, la sal y la pimienta y mezcle. Déjelo hervir.

2 Baje la temperatura y cubra con una tapa. Cocine a fuego lento hasta que las coliflores estén blandas. Retire del fuego y haga puré la coliflor con una licuadora de mano.

3 Mientras tanto, coloque una olla a fuego medio. Añada aceite. Cuando el aceite esté caliente, añada

las cebollas y saltéelas durante un par de minutos. Añada los champiñones y saltee hasta que las cebollas estén ligeramente doradas.

4 Añada la coliflor mezclada. Mezcle bien y deje hervir.

5 Reduzca el calor y cocine a fuego lento durante 10-12 minutos. Si la sopa le parece demasiado espesa, añada un poco más de leche y caliéntela bien.

6 Colóquelo en tazones de sopa individuales y sírvalo caliente.

Gazpacho

Preparación: 15 min	Total: 25 min	Porciones: 4

Ingredientes:

- 4 tomates Roma maduros
- 1 cebolla roja pequeña, pelada y picada
- 1 pepino pequeño, pelado, sin semillas, picado
- ½ pimiento verde pequeño, sin semillas, picado
- ½ campana de pimiento rojo, sin semillas, picado
- 2 dientes de ajo grandes, pelados
- 1 chile rojo, sin semillas, sin tallo
- Jugo de media naranja
- 1 cucharadita de cáscara de naranja, rallada
- 1 cucharada de vinagre de sidra de manzana
- 6 cucharadas de aceite de oliva
- ½ taza de jugo de tomate
- ½ taza de agua fría
- ½ cucharadita de sal
- ¼ cucharadita de pimienta en polvo

Para adornar:

- 1 pepino pequeño, finamente picado
- 1 pimiento rojo pequeño, finamente picado

- 1 cebolla roja, finamente picada

Instrucciones:

1. Coloque una olla a fuego medio. Añada los tomates y hierva. Hervir hasta que la piel empiece a agrietarse. Retírelo del calor. Escurra el agua y vierta agua fría sobre ella.
2. Pele los tomates, córtelos en cuartos y quite las semillas.
3. Mezcle los tomates, los pimientos, el pepino, la cebolla, el chile, el ajo, el agua y la cáscara de naranja en una licuadora hasta que esté suave.
4. Añada aceite de oliva, vinagre, jugo de naranja, jugo de tomate, sal y pimienta. Deje hervir durante unos segundos. Si le gusta la consistencia más fina, entonces añada más jugo de tomate.
5. Refrigere y sirva frío en tazones adornados con pepino, pimiento rojo y cebolla.

Sopa de zanahoria y calabacín

Preparación: 15 min	Total: 55 min	Porciones: 4

Ingredientes:

- 2 zanahorias grandes, peladas y picadas en trozos grandes
- 1 manzana pelada, sin semilla y picada en trozos grandes
- 2 calabacines, pelados, picados en trozos grandes
- 1 cucharada de jengibre fresco, picado
- ½ cucharadita de cúrcuma
- 2 tazas de caldo vegetal
- 1/ 8 cucharadita de canela en polvo
- Sal y pimienta al gusto
- 1 cucharada de aceite de coco
- ½ taza de leche de coco

Instrucciones:

1. Coloca una olla con aceite a fuego medio-alto. Añada las cebollas y saltee hasta que estén translúcidas.

2. Añada el jengibre y saltee durante un par de minutos. Añada el resto de los ingredientes, excepto la leche de coco, y deje que hierva.
3. Reduzca el calor y cocine a fuego lento durante unos 30 minutos. Mezcle con una licuadora de mano.
4. Añada la leche de coco, revuelva bien y sirva.

Sopa de Coliflor

Preparación: 20 min	Total: 45 min	Porciones: 10

Ingredientes:

- 2 cabezas medianas de coliflor, picadas en trozos grandes
- 2 zanahorias grandes, picadas
- 2 cebollas, cortadas en cubitos
- 4 dientes de ajo, picados
- 4 tallos de apio, picados
- 8 tazas de caldo vegetal
- 2 tazas de leche de coco
- 1 cucharada de aceite de coco
- 1 cucharadita de cilantro molido
- 1 cucharadita de cúrcuma
- 1 ½ cucharaditas de comino molido
- 2 cucharadas de eneldo fresco, picado
- Sal al gusto
- Pimienta al gusto

Instrucciones:

1. Coloque una olla a fuego medio-alto. Añada aceite. Cuando el aceite se caliente, agregue las

cebollas, el ajo, las zanahorias y el apio y saltee hasta que las cebollas estén translúcidas.

2. Añada la coliflor y saltéela durante unos 5 minutos.

3. Añada el resto de los ingredientes, excepto el eneldo, y deje que hierva.

4. Baje la temperatura y cubra con una tapa. Cocine a fuego lento hasta que las verduras estén tiernas.

5. Adorne con eneldo y sirva.

Sopa cremosa de tomate sin crema

Preparación: 10 min	Total: 20 min	Porciones: 4

Ingredientes:

- 8 tomates Roma
- 1 taza de tomates secos al sol
- 1 taza de nueces de macadamia crudas
- 2 cucharaditas de sal marina o al gusto
- ½ taza de albahaca fresca
- 1 cucharadita de pimienta blanca o al gusto
- ¼ cucharadita de pimienta negra
- 2 dientes de ajo
- 4 tazas de agua

Instrucciones:

1. Añada todos los ingredientes en una licuadora y mezcle hasta que esté suave.
2. Transfiera el contenido a una olla grande y caliéntelo bien.
3. Sirva caliente.

Sopa agridulce china

Preparación: 10 min	Total: 50 min	Porciones: 3

Ingredientes:

- 3 tazas de caldo de verduras
- 1 taza de champiñones, en rodajas
- ½ lata pequeña de brotes de bambú
- ½ lata pequeña de castañas de agua en lata
- 1 cucharada de salsa de soja
- ¼ cucharadita de pimienta
- 1 cucharadita de salsa picante
- 1 cucharada de vinagre
- 2 dientes de ajo, picados
- ½ taza de cebolletas en rodajas
- 1 cucharada de aceite de chile

Instrucciones:

1. Añada todos los ingredientes excepto las cebolletas y el aceite de chile a una olla grande. Ponga la olla a fuego medio y deje que hierva.
2. Baje la temperatura y cubra con una tapa. Cocine a fuego lento durante unos 20-25 minutos o hasta que las verduras estén tiernas.

3. Añada las cebolletas y deje hervir durante 5 minutos. Pruebe y regule los condimentos si es necesario.

4.Colóquelo en tazones de sopa y sirva.

Capítulo 3: Recetas cetogénicas de ensalada vegana

Ensalada griega

Preparación: 10 min	Total: 12 min	Porciones: 4

Ingredientes:

<u>Para la ensalada:</u>

- 2 pepinos, picados
- 8 tomates, picados
- 1 cebolla roja, en rodajas finas
- 1 ½ tazas de aceitunas Kalamata

<u>Para el aliño al estilo griego:</u>

- ¼ taza de vinagre de vino tinto
- ½ taza de aceite de oliva virgen extra
- 2 cucharadas de jugo de limón fresco
- 1 cucharadita de orégano seco
- Sal marina al gusto
- Polvo de pimienta negra recién molida al gusto

Instrucciones:

1. Agregue los tomates, el pepino y las cebollas rojas a un tazón y mezcle.
2. Para hacer el aliño: Añada todos los ingredientes del aderezo en un recipiente y bata bien.
3. Vierta el aliño sobre la ensalada y mezcle bien.
4. Coloque aceitunas y sirva.

Ensalada de coliflor

Preparación: 10 min	Total: 40 min	Porciones: 4

Ingredientes:

- 2 coliflores, partidas en ramilletes
- 2 cebollas, en rodajas
- ¼ taza de aceite de oliva
- ½ taza de espinaca bebé
- 1/3 taza de vinagre de jerez
- ½ taza de eneldo fresco, cortado
- 1/3 taza de almendras, tostadas, cortadas en rodajas
- Sal al gusto
- Pimienta al gusto

Instrucciones:

1. Añada la coliflor a una fuente para hornear. Espolvoree sal, pimienta y aceite de oliva. Mezcle bien.
2. Precaliente el horno a 350° F durante unos 15 minutos.
3. Añada las cebollas, mézclelas bien y hornee durante otros 15 minutos.

4. Mientras tanto, prepare el aderezo de la siguiente manera: Mezcle el vinagre, la sal y la pimienta. Añada almendras.
5. Añada la coliflor a un tazón. Añada espinacas y eneldo. Vierta el aderezo. Mezcle y sirva.

Ensalada de Limón y Amapola Tahini

Preparación: 10 min	Total: 15 min	Porciones: 2

Ingredientes:

- 7-8 hojas de lechuga
- ½ taza de semillas de girasol o Tahini
- ½ taza de col morada, rallada

Para el aliño:

- 2 cucharadas de jugo de limón
- 2 cucharadas de aceite de oliva virgen extra
- ½ cucharadita de jengibre rallado
- ½ cucharada de semillas de amapola
- 1/8 de cucharadita de sal
- Pimienta al gusto

Instrucciones:

1. Bata todos los ingredientes del aliño en un recipiente. Deje a un lado por un tiempo para que los sabores se fijen.
2. Mezcle en un bol, la col, las semillas de girasol y el aliño.

3. Coloque las hojas de lechuga en una fuente para servir. Coloque la mezcla de col sobre las hojas de lechuga y sirva.

Tabulé de Coliflor

Preparación: 15 min	Total: 16 min	Porciones: 4

Ingredientes:

- 4 tazas de coliflor, rallada o picada finamente
- ¼ taza de hojas de menta fresca, picada
- 1 taza de perejil fresco, picado
- 2 tazas de tomates frescos, picados
- ¼ taza de jugo de limón
- Pimienta al gusto
- Sal al gusto
- ½ taza de aceite de oliva
- 2 cucharadas de ralladura de limón

Instrucciones:

1. Añada todos los ingredientes en un recipiente y revuelva hasta que estén bien combinados.
2. Deje enfriar una hora.
3. Mezcle bien y sirva.

Ensalada Tempeh

Preparación: 20 min	Total: 22 min	Porciones: 4

Ingredientes:

- 2 tazas de Tempeh, en cubos
- 2 palitos de apio, picados
- 1 cebolla, picada
- 2 encurtidos medianos, picados
- ¼ taza de perejil, picado
- 1 ½ cucharadas de salsa de soja
- 2 cucharadas de polvo de curry o al gusto
- 2 dientes de ajo picados
- 2 cucharadas de mostaza

Instrucciones:

1. Vaporice el Tempeh. Deje enfriar por completo.
2. Añada todos los ingredientes en un recipiente grande. Mezcle bien, enfríe un par de horas y sirva.

Ensalada de atún simulada

Preparación: 15 min	Total: 16 min	Porciones: 8

Ingredientes:

- 2 tazas de tofu extra firme, escurrido, prensado en cubos
- ½ taza de zanahorias, finamente picadas
- ½ taza de apio, finamente picado
- 1 cucharadita de polvo de algas marinas
- 2 cucharaditas de jugo de limón
- 1 taza de mayonesa vegana
- 2 cucharaditas de cebolla en polvo
- Sal al gusto
- Pimienta al gusto
- Bocadillos de algas para servir
- Palitos de apio para servir

Instrucciones:

1. Añada todos los ingredientes en un bol y mézclelos bien.
2. Cubra con palitos de apio y aperitivos de algas y sirva.

Ensalada Tailandesa

Preparación: 15 min	Total: 17 min	Porciones: 2

Ingredientes:

- ½ taza de zanahorias, peladas, picadas
- ¼ taza de cilantro, picado
- 1 diente de ajo, picado
- Jugo de ½ un limón
- 1 ½ tazas de col rizada, picada
- 1 taza de col china, picado
- 1 pimiento rojo, picado
- 1 taza de leche de coco fina
- 2 cucharadas de mantequilla de maní cremosa
- ½ cucharadita de salsa Sriracha
- ½ cucharadita de polvo de curry amarillo
- Sal Kosher al gusto

Instrucciones:

1. Para hacer el aliño: Añada el ajo, el jugo de limón, la mantequilla de maní, el polvo de curry y la leche de coco a un tazón y mezcle bien.
2. Mezcle el resto de los ingredientes en un recipiente grande. Luego, añada el aliño.

3.Sirva.

Ensalada de col morada y nuez

Preparación: 10 min	Total: 12 min	Porciones: 4

Ingredientes:

Para la ensalada:

- 8 tazas de col morado, cortado en rebanadas finas
- ½ taza de nueces chinas
- 2 cebolletas, picadas, las partes verdes y blancas

Para el aliño:

- ¼ taza de vinagre
- 2-3 gotas de Stevia líquida
- 2 cucharadas de aceite de oliva
- 2 cucharadas de salsa de soja

Instrucciones:

1. Mezcle en un bol todos los ingredientes del aderezo.
2. Mezcle en un recipiente grande el resto de los ingredientes.
3. Vierta el aliño sobre la ensalada y revuelva.
4. Sirva inmediatamente.

Capítulo 4: Recetas de aperitivos/bocadillos veganos Cetogénicos

Keto Hummus

Preparación: 10 min	Total: 12 min	Porciones: 12

Ingredientes:

- 2 tazas de calabacín, pelado y picado
- ¼ taza de jugo de limón fresco
- 2 dientes de ajo, pelados
- ½ cucharada de comino molido
- 6 cucharadas de Tahini
- 2 cucharadas de aceite de oliva
- 1 cucharadita de sal o al gusto

Para adornar:

- 2 cucharadas de perejil fresco picado
- 1 cucharada de aceite de oliva
- ¼ cucharadita de pimentón

Instrucciones:

1. Añada todos los ingredientes en una licuadora y mezcle hasta que esté suave. Transfiéralo a un tazón.
2. Adorne con perejil y pimentón. Rocíe aceite de oliva en la parte superior y sirva.
3. Una porción es de 2 cucharadas.

Palomitas de Coliflor

Preparación: 10 min	Total: 1 hora. 10 minutos	Porciones: 8

Ingredientes:

- 2 cabezas de coliflor, cortadas en pequeños trozos (aproximadamente una pulgada)
- ½ taza de aceite de oliva
- Sal al gusto
- ½ cucharadita de trozos de pimiento rojo

Instrucciones:

1. Añada el aceite de oliva y la sal en un bol grande. Mezcle bien.
2. Añada los trozos de coliflor y mézclelos hasta que estén bien combinados.
3. Forre una bandeja grande para hornear con papel aluminio. Ponga la coliflor en la bandeja para hornear. Extiéndelo por toda la bandeja.
4. Caliente un horno precalentado a 375° F durante aproximadamente una hora o hasta que la coliflor esté dorada.

Chips de chirivía

Preparación: 10 min	Total: 20 min	Porciones: 6

Ingredientes:

- 3 chirivías medianas, cortadas en rodajas redondas de ¼ pulgadas de grosor
- 3 cucharadas de aceite de oliva virgen extra
- Ajo en polvo (opcional)
- ¼ cucharadita de sal o al gusto
- ¼ polvo de pimienta negra
- ½ cucharadita de pimentón
- Cualquier hierba seca de su elección como el romero o el eneldo (opcional)

Instrucciones:

1. Unte las rodajas de chirivía por ambos lados con aceite de oliva. Coloque las rodajas de chirivía en una bandeja para hornear forrada.
2. Rocíe sal, pimienta, pimentón y hierbas, ajo en polvo si está usando
3. Coloque las rodajas de chirivía en una sola capa.
4. Hornee las rodajas de chirivía en un horno precalentado a 400° F durante 10 minutos o hasta

que esté crujiente. Voltea las chirivías una vez a la mitad de la cocción.

5. Retirar del horno. Enfriar en una rejilla de alambre y sirva.

Nota: Se pueden hacer papas fritas con col rizada o calabacines o papas dulces de manera similar.

Solo varía el tiempo de cocción.

Barras de granola

Preparación: 15 min	Total: 20 min	Porciones: 12

Ingredientes:

- 1½ tazas de nueces y semillas mixtas de su elección
- ½ taza de arándanos secos
- 1 taza de coco rallado sin azúcar
- 2 cucharadas de aceite de coco
- ¼ taza de mantequilla de semillas de girasol
- Gotas de Stevia al gusto
- ¼ cucharadita de extracto de vainilla
- ¼ cucharadita de sal marina
- ½ cucharadita de canela molida

Instrucciones:

1. Forre un plato Pyrex con papel pergamino y déjelo a un lado.
2. Corte la mitad de las nueces en trozos pequeños. Añada el resto de las nueces al procesador de alimentos y pulse hasta que los trozos sean más pequeños que los trozos picados.

3. Añada todas las nueces a un tazón. Agregue los arándanos y el coco rallado, y mezcle bien.

4. Añada el aceite de coco, la mantequilla de girasol, la miel, la vainilla, la sal y la canela a una cacerola pequeña y colóquela a fuego medio-bajo. Cuando empiece a burbujear, retire del fuego.

5. Vierta esta mezcla en el bol de las nueces y revuelva bien. Transfiera todo el contenido al plato preparado. Esparza por todo el plato. Mezcle bien y manténgalo a un lado durante 2 horas.

6. Cubra y colóquelo en el congelador durante una hora.

7. Corte en barras y sirva.

Almendras picantes

Preparación: 5 min	Total: 35 min	Porciones: 12

Ingredientes:

- 3 tazas de almendras
- 1 cucharada de aceite de oliva extra virgen
- 1 ½ cucharadita de comino molido
- 1 ½ cucharaditas de cilantro molido
- 1 cucharadita de chile en polvo
- 1 ½ cucharaditas de polvo de curry (opcional)
- ½ cucharadita de sal marina
- ¼ cucharadita de pimienta de cayena o al gusto

Instrucciones:

1. Coloque las almendras en una fuente para hornear. Añada el resto de los ingredientes al plato y mézclelos bien.
2. Colóquelo en un horno precalentado a 350° F durante unos 30 minutos o hasta que esté listo.
3. Deje enfriar y almacene en un recipiente hermético
Nota: Las almendras pueden ser reemplazadas por nueces de macadamia o cualquier otra nuez de su elección.

Papas fritas de berenjena

Preparación: 10 min	Total: 30 min	Porciones: 6-8

Ingredientes:

- 2 berenjenas medianas, cortadas en rodajas de 1 cm y luego cortadas en tiras de 1 cm
- 2 cucharadas de aceite de oliva
- Sal al gusto
- Pimienta en polvo al gusto
- Ajo en polvo al gusto

Instrucciones:

1. Coloque las tiras de berenjena en una bandeja de hornear. Unte con aceite.
2. Espolvoree sal, ajo en polvo y pimienta.
3. Colóquelo en un horno precalentado a 400° F durante unos 20 minutos o hasta que se dore,
4. Espolvoree más sal, ajo en polvo y pimienta y sirva.

Papas fritas de calabacín ahumado

Preparación: 10 min	Total: 55 min	Porciones: 4-6

Ingredientes:

- 3 calabacines medianos
- Sal al gusto
- 2 cucharadas de aceite de oliva
- 3 cucharaditas de pimentón ahumado o al gusto
- Pimienta en polvo a gusto

Instrucciones:

1. Corte el calabacín en rodajas de ¼ pulgadas de grosor, en forma transversal con una rebanadora o un cuchillo.
2. Coloque los calabacines en un colador en capas, rocíelas con sal y pimienta para que la humedad se escurra.
3. Seque las rebanadas de calabacín con un papel toalla y colóquelas en una bandeja para hornear engrasada.
4. Unte la parte superior de las rodajas de calabacín con aceite. Espolvorea pimentón y pimienta.

5. Colóquele en un horno precalentado a 250° F durante 45 minutos. Apague el horno y deje que las papas fritas permanezcan en el interior durante una hora para que quede crujiente.

6. Transfiera las papas fritas a un contenedor hermético cuando se enfríe.

Wraps de Lechuga

Preparación: 10 min	Total: 13 min	Porciones: 8

Ingredientes:

- 8 hojas de lechuga iceberg
- 1 zanahoria grande, cortada en tiras
- ½ pepino, cortado en fósforos
- ½ taza de Keto hummus
- ¼ cucharadita de pimentón

Instrucciones:

1. Esparza hojas de lechuga en su área de trabajo.
2. Divida y coloque las zanahorias y el pepino sobre las hojas de lechuga. Añada una cucharada de humus. Espolvoree pimentón.
3. Enrolle y sirva.

"Cuñas de patata" de Búfalo

Preparación: 10 min	Total: 55 min	Porciones: 4-6

Ingredientes:

- 4 colinabos medianos, enjuagados, pelados y cortados en trozos
- 1 taza de salsa de alas de búfalo
- 8 cucharadas de mantequilla vegana, derretida
- 1 cucharadita de cebolla en polvo
- 4 cebollas de verdeo, picadas
- 1 cucharadita de sal o sabor
- Pimienta en polvo al gusto

Instrucciones:

1. Añada mantequilla, sal, cebolla en polvo y pimienta negra en polvo a un tazón. Sumerja las cuñas de colinabo y cúbralas bien.
2. Coloque las cuñas en una bandeja de hornear forrada en una capa.
3. Colóquelo en un horno precalentado a 400° F durante unos 30 minutos.
4. Retire del horno y vierta la salsa de alas de búfalo, revuelva y hornee durante otros 15 minutos.

5. Retire del horno, sirva con cebollas de verdeo.

Edamame de Soya y Sésamo

Preparación: 1 min	Total: 5 min	Porciones: 4

Ingredientes:

- 3 tazas de edamame en vainas
- 2 cucharaditas de salsa de soja
- Pimienta al gusto
- Sal al gusto
- 4 cucharadas de aceite de sésamo, tostado

Instrucciones:

1. Coloque una olla con agua a fuego medio. Deje hervir. Añada el edamame y hierva durante 5 minutos.
2. Escurra y colóquelo en un tazón de agua fría. Escurra y deje secar.
3. Coloque una olla a fuego alto. Añada aceite de sésamo. Cuando el aceite esté bien caliente, añada edamame y saltee hasta que esté de color marrón claro.
4. Añada la salsa de soja y cocine hasta que se seque.
5. Agregue sal y una pizca generosa de pimienta. Mezcle bien.
6. Sirva ya sea caliente o frío.

Capítulo 5: Recetas de platos principales veganos Cetogénicos

Arroz de coliflor

Preparación: 10 min	Total: 20 min	Porciones: 4

Ingredientes:

- 2 cabezas de coliflor, cortadas en trozos
- 1 cebolla, finamente picada
- 4 cucharadas de aceite de oliva
- 4 dientes de ajo, picados
- Sal al gusto
- Pimienta en polvo a gusto

Instrucciones:

1. Añada los trozos de coliflor al tazón del procesador de alimentos y mezcle hasta obtener

una textura similar a la del arroz. Alternativamente, ralle la coliflor si es necesario.

2. Coloque una sartén antiadherente grande a fuego medio-alto. Añada aceite. Cuando el aceite esté caliente, añada las cebollas y saltéelas hasta que estén translúcidas. Añada el ajo y saltee durante un minuto hasta que esté listo.

3. Añada el arroz con coliflor y saltéelo durante unos 5-6 minutos. Retírelo del calor.

4. Espolvoree sal y pimienta justo antes de servir.

5. Sirva caliente con una salsa o curry de su elección.

Arroz Mexicano de Coliflor

Preparación: 15 min	Total: 30 min	Porciones: 6

Ingredientes:

- 6 tazas de trozos de coliflor
- 1 cebolla grande, picada
- 2 jalapeños, finamente picados + extra para adornar
- 1 ½ tazas de pimiento, cortado en cubos
- 8 dientes de ajo, picados
- 4 tomates medianos, finamente picados
- 2 cucharaditas de comino molido
- Sal al gusto
- 1 cucharadita de pimentón o chile en polvo
- 2 cucharadas de jugo de lima
- 1 aguacate, pelado, sin semilla, en rodajas
- 2 cucharadas de aceite de oliva
- 2 cucharadas de cilantro fresco picado

Instrucciones:

1. Añada los trozos de coliflor al tazón del procesador de alimentos y mezcle hasta obtener

una textura similar a la del arroz. Alternativamente, ralle la coliflor si es necesario.

2. Coloque una sartén antiadherente grande a fuego medio-alto. Añada aceite. Cuando el aceite esté caliente, añada las cebollas y saltéelas hasta que estén translúcidas. Añada el ajo y los jalapeños y saltéelos durante un minuto hasta que estén listos.

3. Agregue los tomates, el comino, el pimentón y la sal y saltee hasta que los tomates estén blandos.

4. Añada el arroz con coliflor y el pimiento y saltéelo durante unos 5-6 minutos. Retírelo del calor.

5. Divida y sirva en platos. Adorne con cilantro. Rocíe el jugo de limón. Coloque las rebanadas de aguacate encima y sirva.

Wraps de Lechuga Tempeh

Preparación: 10 min	Total: 18 min	Porciones: 8

Ingredientes:

- 2 paquetes de Tempeh, desmenuzado
- 1 cebolla, picada
- 1 pimiento rojo, picado
- 2 cabezas de lechuga de hoja de mantequilla - 8 hojas
- 2 cucharadas de aceite de oliva
- 2 cucharadas de ajo, picado
- 2 cucharadas de salsa de soja baja en sodio
- 2 cucharaditas de ajo en polvo
- 2 cucharaditas de jengibre en polvo
- 2 cucharaditas de cebolla en polvo
- Sal al gusto

Instrucciones:

1. Coloque una olla grande a fuego medio. Añada aceite. Cuando el aceite se caliente, agregue el ajo y saltee hasta que esté fragante.
2. Añada las cebollas, el Tempeh y el pimiento y saltee hasta que las cebollas estén translúcidas.

3. Añada la salsa de soja, el ajo en polvo, el jengibre en polvo, la cebolla en polvo y la sal y cocine durante un par de minutos.
4. Extienda las hojas de lechuga en su área de trabajo. Distribuya la mezcla de Tempeh sobre las hojas de lechuga. Enrolle y sirva.

Bol de Tacos de Jaca y Coliflor

Preparación: 12 min	Total: 22 min	Porciones: 6

Ingredientes:

- 2 latas de jaca joven en agua, escurrida, cortada en trozos más pequeños
- 2 tazas de col rizada congelada
- 1 cucharadita de cebolla en polvo al gusto
- 1 cucharadita de ajo en polvo o al gusto
- 2 cucharadas de aceite de oliva
- 2 cucharadas de condimento para tacos o chile en polvo o al gusto
- 8 tazas de ramilletes de coliflor

Para servir:

- Guacamole
- Queso vegano

Instrucciones:

1. Añada los trozos de coliflor al tazón del procesador de alimentos y mezcle hasta obtener una textura similar a la del arroz. Alternativamente, ralle la coliflor si es necesario.

91

2. Coloque una sartén antiadherente grande a fuego medio-alto. Añada aceite. Cuando el aceite esté caliente, añada las cebollas y saltéelas hasta que estén translúcidas. Añada el ajo y saltee durante un minuto hasta que esté lista.

3. Añada el arroz con coliflor y saltéelo durante unos 5-6 minutos. Retírelo del calor.

4. Divida y sirva en tazones. Cubra con guacamole y queso vegano y sirva.

Tofu crujiente prensado con ajo y menta

Preparación: 15 min	Total: 27 min	Porciones: 2

Ingredientes:

- Paquete de 14 onzas de tofu extra firme
- 2 cucharadas de aceite de oliva virgen extra
- ¼ taza de hojas de menta fresca, picada
- Ralladura de limón ½, finamente rallado
- 2 dientes de ajo grandes
- ¾ cucharadita de sal marina o al gusto
- 2 cucharadas de jugo de limón
- ½ cucharadita de hojuelas de pimiento rojo o al gusto

Instrucciones:

1. Corte el tofu en 2 rebanadas gruesas. Colóquela sobre capas de papel toalla y presione para eliminar el exceso de humedad.
2. Mezcle el resto de los ingredientes en un bol.
3. Añada el tofu y mezcle bien. Deje marinar el tofu durante un mínimo de 30 minutos.
4. Coloque una sartén antiadherente a fuego medio. Retire el tofu del adobo y colóquelo en la sartén.

Cocine hasta que la parte inferior esté dorada. Voltee por ambos lados y cocine el otro lado hasta que se dore.

5. Retírelo del calor y colóquelo en una fuente de servir.
6. Vierta el adobo en la sartén y cocine por un par de minutos.
7. Vierta sobre el tofu cocido y sirva inmediatamente.

Wraps de col

Preparación: 10 min	Total: 20 min	Porciones: 6 -8

Ingredientes:

- 4 tazas de nueces
- 3 cucharaditas de chile en polvo o al gusto
- 14 cucharadita de pimienta de cayena
- 2 cucharadas de comino molido
- 3 cucharaditas de cilantro molido
- 12 hojas grandes de color verde col rizada, desechar los tallos, cortados a 2 pulgadas de la parte inferior de las hojas
- 4 cucharadas de tamari bajo en sodio
- Salsa según sea necesario

Instrucciones:

1. Añada las nueces en el tazón del procesador de alimentos y mezcle hasta que las nueces tengan una textura espesa. Pase la mezcla a un bol y añada las especias y el tamari y mezcle bien.
2. Extienda las hojas de col rizada con el lado claro hacia arriba en su área de trabajo.

95

3. Divida la mezcla entre las hojas. Ponga una cucharada de salsa encima. Doble los lados sobre el relleno y enrolle firmemente.
4. Corte en 2 y sirva con un poco más de salsa.

Dal de Coliflor y Calabaza

Preparación: 15 min	Total: 45 min	Porciones: 4

Ingredientes:

- 1 libra de calabaza o calabaza moscada, pelada y cortada en trozos pequeños
- 1 cebolla mediana, finamente picada
- 1 coliflor de cabeza pequeña, cortada en pequeños ramilletes
- 1 ½ cucharadas de aceite de coco
- 2 dientes de ajo, picados
- ½ cucharada de jengibre rallado
- ½ cucharadita de comino en polvo
- ½ cucharadita de polvo de cúrcuma
- ¼ cucharadita de copos de chile rojo
- 1 cucharadita de polvo de curry suave
- 1 taza de caldo vegetal
- 1 cucharada de jugo de limón
- ½ taza de crema de coco + extra para adornar
- 2 cucharadas de semillas de sésamo + extra para la guarnición
- 2 cucharadas de cilantro fresco picado
- ½ cucharadita de sal o al gusto

Instrucciones:

1. Coloque una sartén grande a fuego medio. Añada aceite de coco. Cuando el aceite se derrita, añada las cebollas y saltee hasta que las cebollas estén ligeramente doradas.
2. Añada calabaza, jengibre y ajo. Saltee durante un par de minutos hasta que esté lista.
3. Añada la cúrcuma, el comino, el polvo de curry y las hojuelas de chile y saltee durante unos segundos.
4. Añada el caldo vegetal, la crema de coco, el jugo de limón, la sal y las semillas de sésamo. Mezcle bien y deje hervir.
5. Baje la temperatura y cubra con una tapa. Cocine a fuego lento durante unos 10 minutos.
6. Mientras tanto, coloque la coliflor en el tazón del procesador de alimentos y mezcle hasta que tenga una textura fina o hasta que tenga una textura parecida al arroz.
7. Añada coliflor. Revuelva, cubra y cocine hasta que esté listo. Triture la coliflor con un pasapurés.
8. Adorne con cilantro, semillas de sésamo y crema de coco.

Bol de fideos con curry cremoso

Preparación: 15 min	Total: 25 min	Porciones: 8

Ingredientes:

- 2 paquetes completos de fideos kanten
- 1 cabeza de coliflor, picada
- 4 zanahorias, en juliana
- 2 pimientos rojos, picados
- 8 tazas de verduras mixtas
- ½ taza de cilantro fresco, picado

Para la salsa cremosa de curry:

- ½ taza de Tahini
- ½ taza de agua
- 4 cucharaditas de polvo de curry
- 1 cucharadita de cúrcuma molida
- 3 cucharaditas de cilantro molido
- 2 cucharaditas de comino molido
- ½ cucharadita de jengibre molido
- 1 cucharadita de pimienta negra
- 2 cucharaditas de sal marina o al gusto
- 4 cucharadas de aceite de aguacate o aceite MCT
- 4 cucharadas de vinagre de sidra de manzana

Instrucciones:

1. Para hacer la salsa de curry: Añada todos los ingredientes de la salsa de curry en una licuadora y bata hasta que esté suave. Déjelo reposar por un momento.
2. Coloque las hojas de fideos en un recipiente grande y vierta agua caliente sobre ellas (no hirviendo, pero que este tibio). Remoje durante unos 5 minutos. Escurra y reserve por un momento.
3. Añada la coliflor, las zanahorias, los pimientos y el cilantro y mezcle bien.
4. Coloque las hojas de la ensalada en platos individuales. Coloque los fideos y las verduras encima.
5. Vierta la salsa cremosa de curry sobre ella y sirva. Se puede enfriar y servir más tarde también.

Lasaña de berenjena

Preparación: 20 min	Total: 1 hora. 30 minutos	Porciones: 8

Ingredientes:

- 3 libras de berenjenas, cortadas en rodajas de 2 milímetros
- 2 tazas de queso mozzarella vegetariano, en rebanadas
- 4 latas (15 onzas cada una) de tomates cortados en cubos, sin sal
- 2 libras de hongos, en rebanadas
- 2 cebollas grandes, cortadas en cubos
- 5-6 dientes de ajo, picados
- 2 cucharadas de aceite de oliva
- 3-4 cucharadas de condimento italiano
- Sal al gusto
- Pimienta al gusto
- Aerosol de cocina

Instrucciones:

1. Para hacer salsa: Coloque una sartén grande con aceite a fuego medio-alto. Añada el ajo y saltee durante un minuto hasta que esté fragante.

101

2. Añada las cebollas y saltéelas hasta que estén translúcidas. Añada los hongos y cocine hasta que se doren. Agregue el resto de los ingredientes excepto la berenjena y el queso. Mezcle bien y deje hervir.

3. Reduzca el calor y cúbralo con una tapa. Cocine a fuego lento durante 8-10 minutos. Revuelva de vez en cuando. Destape y cocine por otros 15 minutos revolviendo ocasionalmente.

4. Forre una bandeja grande rectangular para hornear con papel de aluminio. Roció con spray de cocina. Coloque la mitad de las berenjenas en una sola capa sin sobreponerlas. Esparza la mitad de la salsa sobre ella.

5. Coloque las rebanadas de berenjena restantes sobre la salsa. Esparza el resto de la salsa sobre ella. Cubra con papel aluminio.

6. Colóquelo en un horno precalentado a 325° F durante 30 minutos. Suba la temperatura a 375° F y hornee por otros 30 minutos.

7. Retire del horno. Retire el papel aluminio y coloque las rebanadas de queso por todo el plato. Hornee hasta que el queso se derrita. Deje que se quede en el horno durante 10 minutos antes de servir.

Pan Vegano

Preparación: 15 min	Total: 1 hora. 15 minutos	Porciones: 8

Ingredientes:

- 2 tazas de champiñones, picados
- 1 cebolla roja, cortada en cubitos
- 2 cucharadas de aceite de coco
- 1 taza de semillas de girasol
- 1 taza de harina de almendra finamente molida
- ½ cucharadita de sal de roca del Himalaya
- 4 dientes de ajo, picados
- 2 cucharadas de linaza finamente molida
- 6 cucharadas de agua caliente
- 2 tazas de corazones de cáñamo
- 4 cucharaditas de mezcla de especias de su elección

Instrucciones:

1. Engrase con aceite 2 moldes de pan de tamaño mediano y reserve.
2. Añada la cebolla, el ajo y los champiñones y saltéelos hasta que estén ligeramente dorados. Retire del fuego y deje a un lado.

103

3. Mezcle la linaza molida con 6 cucharadas de agua y déjela a un lado durante 5 minutos.
4. Agregue las semillas de girasol al tazón del procesador de alimentos. Mezcle hasta que se reduzcan de tamaño. Añada los corazones de cáñamo, la harina de almendra, la mezcla de especias y la sal. Mezcle hasta que se combinen bien y los corazones de cáñamo sean más pequeños.
5. Transfiéralo a un tazón. Añada la mezcla de cebollas salteadas en el tazón del procesador de alimentos y mezcle hasta que se queden en pequeños trozos. Transfiéralo al tazón de la mezcla de corazón de cáñamo.
6. Mezcle bien. Añada la mezcla de semillas de lino y siga mezclando. Divida la mezcla en 2 partes y coloque cada una de ellas en los moldes de pan.
7. Colóquelo en un horno precalentado a 350° F durante 40-45 minutos o hasta que un palillo de dientes salga limpio cuando se inserte en el centro.
8. Retire del horno y deje enfriar durante un par de horas. Pase un cuchillo por los bordes del pan y retírelo del molde. Corte y sirva.

Risotto de calabaza y queso cheddar bajo en carbohidratos

Preparación: 15 min	Total: 35 min	Porciones: 6

Ingredientes:

- 1 cebolla pequeña, picada
- 6 tazas de coliflor, en forma de arroz
- 6 onzas de queso cheddar vegano, rallado
- 4 cucharadas de mantequilla vegetariana
- Pimienta al gusto
- Sal al gusto
- 1 taza de puré de calabaza o de calabaza de maní
- 4 cucharaditas de pimentón o al gusto
- ½ taza de vino blanco seco (opcional)

Instrucciones:

1. Coloque una olla grande a fuego medio. Añada la mantequilla vegana y derrítala. Añada la cebolla y saltee hasta que esté translúcida. Añada el pimentón, la sal y la pimienta y revuelva durante unos segundos.

2. Añada el vino si es de su preferencia y revuelva. Añada el puré de calabaza y la coliflor y mezcle bien.
3. Cubra con una tapa y cocine a fuego lento durante 15 minutos o hasta que la coliflor se ablande. Revuelva un par de veces mientras se está cocinando. Pruebe y ajuste el condimento si es necesario.
4. Retírelo del calor. Agregue el queso cheddar vegano y revuelva.
5. Sirva caliente.

Ensalada de zanahoria con triángulos de Tempeh ahumado

Preparación: 15min	Total: 20 min	Porciones: 8

Ingredientes:

- 16 onzas de Tempeh, cortados en triángulos
- 5-6 cucharaditas de tamari o salsa de soja
- 8 tazas de zanahorias, ralladas
- 2 cucharadas de nueces, trituradas
- 2 cebollas pequeñas, cortadas en cubos
- ½ cucharadita de humo líquido (opcional)
- 2 cucharaditas de aceite de oliva extra virgen o aceite de coco virgen
- 2 cucharadas de polvo de curry
- ¼ cucharadita de pimienta en polvo o al gusto
- ½ cucharadita de cúrcuma molida
- 4 cucharadas de tahín
- 1 taza de perejil de hoja plana, finamente picado, + extra para adornar
- ½ taza de jugo de limón
- ½ cucharadita de pimienta de cayena o al gusto

- Sal al gusto

Instrucciones:

1. Coloque una sartén a fuego alto. Añada aceite. Cuando se caliente el aceite, añada Tempeh, tamari y humo líquido.
2. Cocine hasta que todo el líquido se absorba y los bordes se doren. Voltee el Tempeh frecuentemente mientras se está cocinando.
3. Añada la nuez y la pimienta y mezcle bien. Retire del calor y cúbralo. Déjelo a un lado por un tiempo.
4. Mezcle el resto de los ingredientes en un tazón y divídalos en platos individuales. Coloque el Tempeh encima y sirva.

Shiritaki "Alfredo" con espinacas

Preparación: 5 min	Total: 13 min	Porciones: 4

Ingredientes:

- 2 paquetes de fideos Shiritaki, escurridos, enjuagados
- 2 tazas de espinacas congeladas
- 4 onzas de queso crema vegano
- Sal al gusto
- Pimienta al gusto
- ½ cucharadita de ajo en polvo
- 2 cucharadas de aceite de oliva
- Leche de almendras según sea necesario

Instrucciones:

1. Añada todos los ingredientes en una sartén. Coloque la sartén a fuego medio. Agregue la leche de almendras según sea necesario y revuelva. Caliente bien la mezcla.
2. Transfiera a los tazones y sirva.

Vegan Keto Lo Mein

Preparación: 10 min	Total: 20 min	Porciones: 4

Ingredientes:

- 2 paquetes de fideos de algas
- 2 tazas de espinacas congeladas
- 1 taza de edamame sin cáscara
- ½ taza de zanahorias, en juliana
- ½ taza de champiñones, rebanados

Para la salsa:

- 4 cucharadas de tamari o salsa de soja
- 1 cucharadita de jengibre molido
- ½ cucharadita de salsa Sriracha
- 2 cucharadas de aceite de sésamo
- 1 cucharadita de ajo en polvo

Instrucciones:

1. Remoje los fideos de algas en un tazón de agua durante un tiempo. Escurra y déjelos a un lado.

2. Para hacer salsa: Coloque una olla a fuego medio-bajo. Añada todos los ingredientes de la salsa en la cacerola y caliéntelos.
3. Cuando la salsa esté caliente, añada los fideos y mézclelos bien. Añada un poco de agua si lo desea para que la mezcla no esté muy seca.
4. Cocine hasta que los fideos estén suaves. Retírelo del calor.
5. Divida y sirva en tazones.

Tofu picante de almendras

Preparación: 10 min	Total: 30 min	Porciones: 4

Ingredientes:

- 2 paquetes de tofu firme o tofu extra firme
- 4 cucharadas de salsa de soja
- 4 cucharadas de agua
- ½ cucharadita de cebolla en polvo
- ½ cucharadita de ajo en polvo
- ½ cucharadita de pimentón
- Sal al gusto
- Pimienta al gusto
- ½ cucharadita de copos de chile
- 2 cucharadas de semillas de sésamo, divididas
- 2 cucharaditas de aceite de sésamo
- 2 cucharadas de aceite de coco
- 4 cucharadas de salsa de chile verde
- ¼ taza de almendras, en rodajas
- Brócoli al vapor para servir

Instrucciones:

1. Coloque el tofu en toallas de papel. Coloque una sartén pesada sobre el tofu para drenar el exceso de humedad. Corte en cubos.
2. Coloque una sartén a fuego alto. Añada aceite de coco. Cuando el aceite se calienta, agregue el tofu y saltee hasta que se dore.
3. Añada las almendras y cocine por un par de minutos. Añada el resto de los ingredientes excepto ½ cucharada de semillas de sésamo y cocine hasta que se seque.
4. Coloque el brócoli al vapor en tazones. Ponga el tofu encima. Rocíe aceite de sésamo sobre él. Espolvoree el resto de las semillas de sésamo encima y sirva.

Pad Thai bajo en carbohidratos

Preparación: 10 min	Total: 13 min	Porciones: 2

Ingredientes:

- ½ bolsa de fideos de algas
- 1 cebolla blanca pequeña
- 2 dientes de ajo, pelados
- 4 cucharadas de mantequilla de maní natural
- 2 cucharadas de salsa de soja o tamari o aminos líquidos
- 1 cucharadita de copos de pimiento rojo
- 2 cucharadas de jugo de lima
- 1 cucharada de semillas de sésamo, tostadas
- 2 cucharadas de cebolletas, picadas
- 2 cucharadas de cilantro picado
- Sal al gusto
- Pimienta en polvo a gusto

Instrucciones:

1. Añada los fideos de algas a un tazón de agua y déjelos en remojo durante un tiempo.
2. Añada la mantequilla de maní, la cebolla, el tamari, el jugo de limón, el ajo, las hojuelas de

pimienta, la pimienta y la sal en una licuadora y mezcle hasta que quede suave y cremoso.

3. Escurra los fideos y colóquelos en un recipiente grande. Vierta la mezcla de mantequilla de maní sobre ella y mezcle bien.

4. Espolvoree semillas de sésamo, cebolletas y cilantro y sirva.

Masa de pizza vegetariana

Preparación: 5 min	Total: 35 min	Porciones: 4

Ingredientes:

- 1 taza de semillas de lino enteras, finamente molidas
- 4 cucharadas de polvo de psyllium
- ½ taza de queso crema vegano
- 2 cucharaditas de polvo de hornear
- 2 cucharaditas de ajo en polvo
- 1 cucharadita de sal o al gusto
- 1 taza de agua

Para la cobertura:

- Salsa para pizza o pesto (Keto amigable)
- Queso vegano según se requiera
- Verduras de su elección, en rodajas

Instrucciones:

1. Añada todos los ingredientes secos en un bol y mézclelos bien. Añada el queso crema vegano y mezcle bien.
2. Agregue agua, poco a poco y mezcle bien para formar la masa.

3. Divida la masa en 2 y darle forma de 2 bolas. Colóquelo en una bandeja de hornear. Aplane para dar forma de una pizza.
9. Colóquelo en un horno precalentado a 350° F durante unos 25 minutos. Voltee los lados y hornee por 5 minutos más
4. Retire del horno y esparza la salsa sobre él. Cubra con verduras y finalmente con queso vegano.
5. Colóquelo de nuevo en el horno. Hornee durante unos 10-15 minutos.
6. Corte en trozos y sirva.

Ultimate Keto Falafel

Preparación: 15 min	Total: 45 min	Porciones: 5

Ingredientes:

- 1 taza de corazones de cáñamo
- 2 cucharadas de perejil fresco picado
- 1 cebolla pequeña, picada
- 2 cucharadas de cilantro fresco picado
- 1 cucharadita de comino molido
- 2 cucharaditas de harina de lino mezcladas con 4 cucharaditas de agua
- 2 cucharaditas de polvo de hornear
- 4 dientes de ajo
- Sal al gusto
- Aceite de coco o aceite de oliva para freír

Para servir:

- 5 tazas de lechuga en rodajas
- 1 pepino pequeño, en rodajas finas
- 1 tomate, en rodajas finas

Instrucciones:

1. Añada todos los ingredientes excepto la mezcla de linaza en el procesador de alimentos y mezcle hasta que estén bien combinados.
2. Añada la mezcla de semillas de lino y mezcle de nuevo. Divida la mezcla en 10 porciones iguales. Forme cada uno de ellos en falafel.
3. Coloque una sartén antiadherente a fuego medio. Añade una cucharada de aceite. Cuando se caliente el aceite, coloque los falafeles sobre él (cocínelo por partes).
4. Cocine hasta que la parte inferior esté dorada. Voltee por ambos lados y cocine hasta que se dore.
5. Ponga una taza de lechuga en 5 platos de servir. Coloque 2 falafel en cada plato. Cubrir con rodajas de tomate y pepino. Servir con Keto hummus.

Rollos de calabacín con coliflor y puré de brócoli

Preparación: 20 min	Total: 55 min	Porciones: 5

Ingredientes:

- 3 calabacines grandes
- 2 cebollas, finamente picadas
- 1 bloque de queso vegano
- 2 pimientos, finamente picados
- 8 dientes de ajo, finamente picados + extra para la parte superior
- 2 cucharadas de pesto
- Sal al gusto
- Pimienta al gusto
- 1 cucharada de aceite de oliva + extra para lloviznar
- 1 coliflor de cabeza mediana, cortado en trozos
- 1 brócoli de cabeza mediana, cortado en trozos
- 2 cucharadas de mantequilla vegana

Instrucciones:

1. Corte 2 de los calabacines en tiras. Colóquelo en un plato grande y espolvoree sal sobre él. Deje los calabacines para después.

2. Cortar el queso vegano en tiras de casi el mismo tamaño que el calabacín. Colóquelo a un lado.
3. Picar el tercer calabacín en pequeños trozos finos.
4. Coloque una sartén a fuego medio. Añada aceite. Cuando el aceite esté caliente, agregue las cebollas y el ajo y saltee hasta que estén ligeramente dorados. Añada los trozos finos de calabacín y pimienta y saltéelos hasta que estén suaves. Añada el pesto. Mezcle bien y retírelo del fuego.
5. Las tiras de calabacín ya se habrían ablandado por la sal.
6. Coloque las tiras de calabacín en su área de trabajo. Esparza el relleno de calabacín sobre las tiras. Coloque las tiras de queso vegano sobre él. Enróllelo firmemente y sujételo con palillos de dientes. Colóquelo en una bandeja de hornear.
7. Espolvoree ajo sobre los rollos. Rocíe un poco de aceite.
8. Colóquelo en un horno precalentado a 350° F durante unos 20- 25 minutos.
9. Mientras tanto, haga el puré de coliflor y brócoli de la siguiente manera: Cocine la coliflor y el brócoli hasta que estén muy blandos.
10. Triture la coliflor y el brócoli con un pasapurés. Añada la mantequilla vegana, sal y pimienta y mezcle bien.
11. Sirva los rollos con puré.

Tofu con salsa tailandesa de coco y maní

Preparación: 5 min	Total: 45 min	Porciones: 4-6

Ingredientes:

- 8 tazas de vegetales mixtos (Keto amigable) de su elección (opcional)
- ½ taza + 2 cucharadas de aceite de coco, divididas
- 2 bloques de tofu firme (alrededor de ¾ libra cada uno)
- 6 dientes de ajo, picados
- 2 chalotas, finamente picadas
- 2 cucharadas de jengibre fresco, rallado
- Pimienta al gusto
- Sal al gusto
- 4 cucharaditas de comino molido
- 2/3 taza de mantequilla de maní o mantequilla de almendra o mantequilla de marañón
- 2 cucharaditas de pimiento rojo triturado
- 1 taza de leche de coco
- 3 cucharadas de tamari o salsa de soja
- Jugo de 2 limas
- 2 cucharaditas de pasta de curry rojo tailandés vegetariana
- ½ taza de cilantro fresco

Instrucciones:

1. Coloque el tofu sobre toallas de papel. Coloque una sartén de fondo grueso sobre ella para drenar el exceso de humedad. Cortar en cuadrados o triángulos de 1 pulgada.
2. Mezcle en un plato grande, ½ taza de aceite, ajo, comino y pimienta. Añada las rebanadas de tofu y mézclelas hasta que estén bien cubiertas. Deje a un lado por un tiempo para marinar.
3. Coloque una sartén a fuego lento. Añada el aceite y caliéntelo. Añada chalota, jengibre, chile rojo triturado. Cocine por unos minutos hasta que esté suave.
4. Añada mantequilla de maní, jugo de limón, leche de coco, tamari y pasta de curry rojo. Mezcle bien y cocine por 10-15 minutos. Revuelva un par de veces mientras se está cocinando.
5. Añada más agua si encuentra la salsa muy espesa. Retírelo del calor y manténgalo caliente.
6. Saltee las verduras en una sartén con el aceite restante.
7. Coloque una sartén a fuego medio. Añada la mezcla de tofu y cocine hasta que se dore.
8. Coloque el tofu con las verduras salteadas en platos individuales. Vierta la salsa encima.
9. Adorne con cilantro y sirva.

Cigkofte Vegano

Preparación: 20 min	Total: 20 min	Porciones: 4

Ingredientes:

- 1 ½ tazas de harina de almendra
- 6 cucharadas de lino molido
- 1 ½ tazas de nueces finamente molidas
- 4 cucharaditas de pimentón
- 4 cucharaditas de menta seca o 4 cucharadas de menta fresca, finamente picada
- 4 cucharaditas de ajo en polvo o 4 dientes de ajo, prensados
- 2 cucharaditas de perejil seco o 2 cucharadas de perejil fresco, finamente picado
- ½ cucharadita de pimienta en polvo o al gusto
- 1 cucharadita de hojuelas de chile
- 6 cucharadas de agua
- 6 cucharadas de puré de tomate

Para servir:

- Hojas de lechuga según sea necesario
- Jugo de limón
- Hojas de menta fresca, picadas

- Perejil fresco, picado

Instrucciones:

1. Añada todos los ingredientes en un recipiente y tritúrelos con un tenedor hasta que se forme una masa gruesa. Es posible que necesite hacer más puré hasta que se forme la masa. Puede que lleve un tiempo en hacerlo.
2. Tome unas 2 cucharadas de la masa y enróllela. Colóquelo en su puño y presione ligeramente para que sus dedos hagan mella en la masa. Colóquelo en un plato.
3. Repita con la masa restante.
4. Sirva sobre las hojas de lechuga. Adorne con menta y perejil. Espolvoree el jugo de limón. Enrolle y sirva.

Moussaka Vegana

Preparación: 20 min	Total: 1 hora y 20 minutos	Porciones: 5-6

Ingredientes:

Para la capa de berenjena:

- 4 berenjenas, cortadas finamente a lo largo en rodajas de ¼ pulgadas de grosor
- 4 cucharadas de aceite de oliva
- 1 cucharada de sal

Para la salsa de tomate:

- 5 onzas de nueces mixtas, finamente picadas
- 2 cucharadas de aceite de oliva
- 2 cucharadas de salsa de soja
- 1 pimiento rojo, picado
- 1 pimiento amarillo, picado
- 10 dientes de ajo, picados
- 2 latas (14 onzas cada una) de tomates cortados en cubos
- ½ cucharadita de nuez moscada molida
- ½ cucharadita de pimienta recién molida

Para la crema de almendras:

126

- 1 taza de almendras, remojadas en agua durante la noche, peladas
- 2 dientes de ajo pequeños
- 2 cucharaditas de vinagre
- ¼ cucharaditas de pimienta recién molida
- 1 taza de agua
- ¼ cucharaditas de sal

Instrucciones:

1. Espolvoree sal sobre las rodajas de berenjena y colóquelas en un colador durante unos 30 minutos.
2. Enjuague y exprima el exceso de humedad de las berenjenas.
3. Coloque un papel aluminio en una bandeja de hornear grande. Coloque las rodajas de berenjena en una sola capa. Unte con aceite.
4. Colóquelo en un horno precalentado a 390° F durante unos 10 minutos o hasta que se dore.
5. Retire del horno y deje enfriar.
6. Mientras tanto, haga la salsa de la siguiente manera: Coloque una sartén a fuego medio. Añada todos los ingredientes de la salsa en ella y deje hervir.
7. Baje el fuego y cocine a fuego lento durante 8-10 minutos.
8. Mientras tanto, haga la crema de almendras de la siguiente manera: Añada todos los ingredientes de

la crema de almendras en una licuadora y bata hasta que esté suave.

9. Para el montaje: utilice una fuente de hornear. Coloque capas alternas de berenjena y salsa de tomate con salsa de tomate como última capa.

10. Vierta la crema de almendras encima.

11. Colóquelo en un horno precalentado a 390° F durante unos 25-30 minutos

Boloñesa picante de hongos y nueces

Preparación: 10 min	Total: 45 min	Porciones: 12

Ingredientes:

- 2 cebollas grandes, finamente picadas
- 2 libras de champiñones, cortados por la mitad, en tiras finas
- 4 tomates ciruela, picados
- 4 dientes de ajo grandes, finamente picados
- 4 latas (14 onzas cada una) de tomates pelados y picados
- 2 tazas de nueces, finamente picadas
- 2 cucharadas de pasta de tomate
- 4 cucharadas de vinagre de manzana
- 2 cucharadas de albahaca seca
- 2 cucharadas de orégano seco
- 2 cucharaditas de pimentón
- 2 cucharaditas de comino molido
- Pimienta al gusto
- Sal al gusto
- Hojuelas de chile rojo al gusto
- 4 cucharadas de aceite de oliva
- Queso parmesano vegano para adornar

Instrucciones:

1. Coloque una olla a fuego medio. Añada aceite. Cuando el aceite se caliente, agregue las cebollas y el ajo y saltee hasta que las cebollas estén translúcidas.
2. Añada los champiñones y saltéelos durante 7-8 minutos. Cuando los champiñones estén secos, añada todas las especias, pasta de tomate, vinagre, albahaca y orégano y mezcle bien.
3. Añada los tomates enlatados y picados y revuelva.
4. Baje el fuego y cocine por unos 20 minutos. Añada las nueces y cocine por 5 minutos más.
5. Sirva con una guarnición de queso parmesano vegano.

Capítulo 7: Recetas cetogénicas de postres vegetarianos

Pudín de chocolate

Preparación: 10 min	Total: 12 min	Porciones: 6

Ingredientes:

- 1 aguacate maduro, pelado, sin semilla, picado
- ½ taza de leche de coco con toda la grasa
- ¼ taza de coco rallado
- 2 cucharadas de polvo de algarroba
- 2 higos secos, picados
- ¼ taza de cacao en polvo
- 2 cucharadas de café instantáneo
- 2 cucharadas de polvo de proteína vegana con sabor a vainilla
- 3 cucharadas de avellanas
- ½ cucharadita de canela molida
- Una gran pizca de sal

Instrucciones:

131

1. Mezcle la leche de coco y el aguacate en una licuadora hasta que esté suave.
2. Añada el resto de los ingredientes excepto el coco y las avellanas. Mezcle hasta que esté suave.
3. Añada el coco y las avellanas y mezcle durante unos segundos hasta que la avellana se rompa en trozos más pequeños.
4. Transfiera la mezcla a tazones, deje enfriar y sirva.

Keto Fudge Super Fácil

Preparación: 2 min	Total: 10 min	Porciones: 4-6

Ingredientes:

- 1 taza de mantequilla de coco o cualquier otra mantequilla de nuez o maná
- 4 onzas de chocolate sin azúcar o 4 onzas de chocolate de panadería y 30 gotas de Stevia

Instrucciones:

1. Coloque una hoja de papel encerado en un recipiente.
2. Añada el chocolate y la mantequilla de coco en una olla y colóquela a fuego lento. Cocine hasta que esté bien combinado. Revuelva con frecuencia.
3. Viértalo en el recipiente preparado. Colóquelo en el refrigerador hasta que esté listo.
4. Corte en cuadrados y sirva.

Mousse de fresa

Preparación: 10 min	Total: 12 min	Porciones: 12

Ingredientes:

- 3 tazas de fresas, en rodajas
- 3 tazas de tofu firme, escurrido, desmenuzado
- Edulcorante de su elección (Swerve o gotas de Stevia)
- Unas cuantas fresas, cortadas para servir

Instrucciones:

1. Mezcle las fresas. Añada el tofu y el edulcorante y mezcle hasta que esté suave.
2. Colóquelos en tazones individuales y refrigérelo durante unas horas antes de servirlo.

Galletas de azúcar veganas Keto

Preparación: 15 min	Total: 35 min	Porciones: 10

Ingredientes:

- 4 onzas de queso crema vegano
- 2-3 cucharadas de Swerve o eritritol
- 6 cucharadas de harina de coco
- ½ cucharadita de extracto de almendra
- ½ cucharadita de extracto de vainilla

Instrucciones:

1. Añada el queso crema, la vainilla y el extracto de almendras en un recipiente y bata hasta que esté cremoso.
2. Agregue la harina de coco y mézclela para formar una masa dura.
3. Coloque entre 2 papeles de cera y enrolle. Córtelas con un cortador de galletas.
4. Colóquelo en una bandeja de hornear. Hornee en un horno precalentado a 350° F durante unos 20 minutos o hasta que los bordes tengan un color marrón dorado.

5. Retire del horno y deje enfriar completamente antes de servir.

Muffins de jengibre con cetona vegana

Preparación: 20 min	Total: 40 min	Porciones: 10

Ingredientes:

- 2 cucharadas de semillas de lino molidas
- 2 cucharadas de vinagre de sidra de manzana
- 4 cucharadas de mezcla de especias de pan de jengibre
- 2 cucharaditas de extracto de vainilla
- ¾ taza de leche de almendras o de coco
- 1 taza de mantequilla de maní
- 2 cucharaditas de polvo de hornear
- 3-4 cucharadas de desvío o al gusto
- 1/8 de cucharadita de sal

Instrucciones:

1. Mezcle en un recipiente, las semillas de lino, el viraje, la sal, la vainilla, la especia de pan de jengibre, la leche de almendras y deje reposar durante 10 minutos.

2. Añada la mantequilla de maní y el polvo de hornear y mezcle bien.
3. Viértalo en moldes de muffins forradas.
4. Coloque los moldes en un horno precalentado a 350° F durante unos 20 minutos o hasta que un palillo de dientes salga limpio cuando se inserte en el centro.
5. Deje enfriar completamente antes de servir.

Rebanada de dulce de leche y chocolate sin hornear

Preparación: 10 min	Total: 30 min	Porciones: 4 - 6

Ingredientes:

Para el dulce de leche:

- 1 taza de mantequilla de marañón o cualquier otra mantequilla de nueces o maná
- 4 onzas de chocolate sin azúcar o 4 onzas de chocolate para panadería y 30 gotas de Stevia
- 1 cucharadita de extracto de vainilla
- Una pizca de sal
- ¾ taza de hojuelas de almendra, tostados

Para la capa de chocolate:

- ½ taza de aceite de coco
- ¼ taza de polvo de cacao crudo
- 2 cucharadas de desvío
- ¼ taza de leche de coco
- 2 cucharaditas de extracto de vainilla

Instrucciones:

1. Ponga una hoja de papel encerado en un recipiente.
2. Añada el chocolate y la mantequilla de coco en una olla y colóquela a fuego lento. Cocine hasta que esté bien combinado. Revuelva con frecuencia. Añada la vainilla y revuelva.
3. Viértalo en el recipiente. Colóquelo en el refrigerador hasta que esté listo.
4. Mientras tanto, coloque todos los ingredientes, excepto el cacao para la capa de chocolate, en una olla. Cuando esté bien mezclado, agregue el cacao en polvo y bata bien hasta que esté suave. Retírelo del calor.
5. Vierta la salsa de chocolate sobre el dulce de leche. Extienda la parte superior con una espátula. Espolvoree las hojuelas de almendra restantes. Refrigere durante 4-5 horas antes de servir. Corte en cuadrados y sirva.

Mini pastel de calabaza con mantequilla de maní baja en carbohidratos

Preparación: 15 min	Total: 40 min	Porciones: 8

Ingredientes:

Para la corteza:

- ½ taza de aceite de coco
- 2 cucharadas de semillas de lino remojadas en 6 cucharadas de agua (llamadas huevos de lino)
- ¾ taza de harina de coco

Para el relleno:

- 2 cucharadas de semillas de lino remojadas en 6 cucharadas de agua
- ½ taza de mantequilla de maní
- ½ desvío de taza o eritritol
- 1 taza de puré de calabaza
- 2 cucharaditas de canela molida

Instrucciones:

1. Mezcle los ingredientes de la corteza en un bol. Tome 8 mini moldes para pastel. Divida la mezcla en los moldes y colóquelas en los moldes.

141

2. Mezcle en un bol todos los ingredientes del relleno. Divida y extienda sobre la corteza.
3. Colóquelo en un horno precalentado a 350° F durante unos 20 minutos.
4. Retire del horno y deje enfriar completamente antes de servir.

Pudín de Chía de Chocolate

Preparación: min 10 min	Total: 45 min	Porciones: 2

Ingredientes:

- ½ cucharadas de semillas de chía
- ½ taza de leche de almendras o leche de soya, sin azúcar
- ½ cucharada de proteína de chocolate vegetariana en polvo o cacao en polvo
- 2 cucharadas de frambuesas, frescas o congeladas
- ½ cuchara de mesa vira si está usando cacao en polvo

Instrucciones:

1. Mezcle la leche de almendra y la proteína de chocolate vegano en polvo con un batidor o un tenedor.
2. Añada las semillas de chía y mézclalas bien. Déjelas a un lado por 5-7 minutos. Mezcle de nuevo.
3. Deje reposar la mezcla durante ½ una hora en el refrigerador.
4. Cubra con frambuesas y sirva.

Brownies de Proteína Keto Vegana

Preparación: 15 min	Total: 40 min	Porciones: 16

Ingredientes:

- 3 tazas de agua caliente
- ½ taza de cacao en polvo, sin azúcar
- 1 taza de mantequilla de maní
- ½ desvío de taza o eritritol
- 4 cucharaditas de polvo de hornear
- 4 cucharadas de proteína de chocolate vegetariana en polvo
- ¼ taza de harina de coco

Instrucciones:

1. Bata el agua y la mantequilla de maní en un tazón.
2. Mezcle el resto de los ingredientes en otro tazón. Añada esto a la mezcla de mantequilla de maní y mezcle hasta que esté bien combinado.
3. Viértalo en una bandeja de hornear engrasada.
4. Coloque la mezcla en un horno precalentado a 350° F durante unos 20 minutos.

5. Retire del horno y deje enfriar completamente antes de servir.
6. Corte y sirva.

Bolas de proteína de arándano con nuez

Preparación: 10 min	Total: 20 min	Porciones: 8

Ingredientes:

- 8 ciruelas pasas, sin semillas
- 1 taza de fresas frescas, picadas
- 1 taza de nueces de macadamia, sin sal, tostadas
- 2 tazas de nueces o almendras
- 1 taza de coco rallado, sin azúcar
- 4 cucharadas de aceite de coco, derretido

Instrucciones:

1. Coloque las ciruelas pasas en el tazón de la procesadora de alimentos y mezcle hasta que estén suaves.
2. Añada nueces o almendras y nueces de macadamia. Siga mezclando hasta que las nueces estén finamente picadas.
3. Con el procesador de alimentos en funcionamiento, vierta lentamente el aceite de coco derretido. Deje que el procesador de alimentos funcione hasta que la mezcla esté bien combinada.

4. Transfiera la mezcla a un tazón. Añada las fresas y mezcle bien para formar la masa. Forme la masa en pequeñas bolas.
5. Coloque el coco rallado en un plato. Enrolle las bolas en el coco rallado y colóquelas en otro plato.
6. Refrigere las bolas hasta que estén listas para servir. Mantenga las bolas que no utilice refrigeradas en un recipiente hermético. Puede durar de 4 a 5 días cuando se refrigera.

Helado vegano de mantequilla de maní con chocolate bajo en carbohidratos

Preparación: 15 min	Total: 17 min + tiempo de congelación	Porciones: 8 - 12

Ingredientes:

- 4 aguacates Hass grandes, pelados, sin semilla, picados
- ½ taza de mantequilla de maní
- ½ taza de cacao en polvo, sin azúcar
- 20 gotas de Stevia o al gusto

Instrucciones:

1. Añada todos los ingredientes en una licuadora y mezcle hasta que esté suave. Viértalo en un contenedor seguro y congélelo durante 4-5 horas o hasta que esté listo.
2. Retire y sirva.

Paletas de Fresa y Lima

Preparación: 10 min	Total: 12 min + tiempo de congelación	Porciones: 5 - 6

Ingredientes:

- 20 fresas medianas y grandes
- Ralladura de 2 limas
- ¼ taza de agua

Instrucciones:

1. Añada todos los ingredientes en una licuadora y mezcle hasta que esté suave.
2. Viértalo en los moldes de paletas y congélelo.
3. Retírelos del molde y sirva.

Conclusión

Le agradezco una vez más por haber elegido este libro y espero que lo haya pasado bien al leerlo. El objetivo principal de este libro era enseñarle los fundamentos de la dieta cetogénica y darte recetas sencillas.

Todas las recetas han sido probadas y seguramente lo dejaran sorprendido. Sin embargo, no se limiten solo a estas recetas y hagan algunas de las suyas.

Puede ampliar el menú y cambiar libremente entre las recetas de la comida y la cena. También puede cambiar los ingredientes y crear platos interesantes.

Recuerde que la cetogénica no es una dieta de moda y requerirá que la convierta en una elección de estilo de vida. Una vez que empiece a utilizarlo, tendrá que hacer el esfuerzo de mantenerlo de por vida.

¡Espero que aproveche todos los beneficios que proporciona la dieta!

¡Buena suerte!

I was making less than $3 an hour. "You don't have to ask that," he said. "Just keep it ... reasonable."

I walked behind the counter to grab a bag and to throw out the wrapper to the licorice, which I'd already devoured in two huge mouth-filling bites.

I glanced over at Dad and Samantha, filling a script for someone with strep throat. Samantha was wearing her long brown hair down, even though sometimes, when she wanted to look older and more professional, she pulled it up and put it in a knot. My father was the same height as her. They worked quietly.

I thought of asking her what she'd said about me, but I didn't want to interrupt. She might be counting the pills with him.

Most girls in my school were wearing jeans now, or jumpers, or something a little fancier when they had someplace to go after school. The school had instituted "Dress Up Day" weekly on Fridays, as some sort of trade off for having loosened the dress code to allow for jeans and other things. Not only did few people respond by dressing up on Fridays as you were supposed to, a fair number of guys got in trouble for pulling girls' dresses up, reminding them, "It's 'Dress-Up Day' ... Get it? 'Dress-UP Day!'"

The girls smacked them, and the guys got after-school detention or a call home. The next week, the whole game would start again. Sometimes with different guys, but usually the same ones. The dumb ones.

So no one wanted to wear anything but jeans now. And we all looked like the teenagers on TV and in *Life* Magazine, but not like San Francisco hippies. We looked like suburban kids who were tired of being in school all week, and who were absolutely not interested in honoring the nifty ideas of the school administrators, who still looked like they had just emerged from 1953.

Looking at Samantha, though, I could tell that there was some sort of effort there to not look like who she actually was – a high schooler a year older than I was. She didn't wear jeans to the pharmacy, and she didn't wear dresses. She wore some sort of slim professional looking pants, along with a white blouse. With her hair laying long onto her back and a studious look on her face, I realized she had projected herself into something else: a woman. A young woman, but a woman.

She must have sensed me staring at her. "Hi, Jerry. I don't know if I told you that I had a sister, Carly. I think she's a year younger than you. What grade are you in again?"

"I'm a junior," I croaked, clearing my throat and trying to sound confident, or whatever a junior was supposed to sound like.

"She's in tenth," Samantha said. "She'd love to meet you; she asked me if you had a girlfriend. You don't have a girlfriend, do you?"

I stood there like a deer in the headlights. It depended on what you defined as a girlfriend. Kendra and I had been best friends since seventh grade. Maybe more than friends?

"No," I said. "I don't."

"Good!" Samantha said. "That's what I told her!"

"How did you know?" I asked.

"Your dad!" she said, laughing. He glanced over at her, and they shared the moment. "How else would I know?"

She suddenly grabbed a prescription label out of the printer, slapped it on the amber bottle, showed it to my father, who read it and nodded. Samantha put it quickly into a small bag, stapling a receipt to the top of it, and placing it in a box for pickup in one swift movement. "She's got a horse," she said. "My sister. His name is Zeus. You like horses?"

"I… um … yeah," I said.

"You should go over and meet him! She'd love to show you and give you a ride. Zeus is real good with beginners."

And with that, I was standing there, almost blushing.

Carly was going to give me a ride.

"Do you want to go? What should I tell her?"

"Could I bring my camera? And take pictures?" I asked. I'd never taken a picture of a horse before. Or of Carly.

"Why not? Is next Tuesday good? Just go there after school and then she can ride you to work here."

"On Montauk Highway? There are cars all over!"

"Zeus is used to them, and there's plenty of space for him on the side of the road. She does it all the time."

Tuesday couldn't come fast enough. I rode my bike all the way to Carly's house, which was only seven miles from my high school. I brought my camera and two rolls of black-and-white film, thirty-six exposures each. I wasn't sure I really wanted or needed seventy-two pictures of a horse.

Carly came to the door, and I was shocked. She was a younger-looking version of Samantha, but even better looking. She wore a baggy Connetquot High School sweatshirt over exceptionally tight jeans that had holes on the front legs in different spots and she made it look like something a fashion model would wear. She laughed, looked down, gestured to them, and said, "I'm sorry, I look hideous, I was just out feeding Zeus, I should've thought…"

Carly and Samantha's mother was home; she was a plain-looking woman who'd clearly gotten ready for me and greeted me with way more excitement than was called for, having set out milk and Oreos at the kitchen table, so we could all talk and get to know each other.

"I feel like I know so much about you from your father!" her mother said. "What a nice man. He's so good to

Samantha."

I didn't know what to say, so I said, "He ... works a lot of hours."

"And Samantha tells me you are helping out there, too."

"After school some days," I said. "And every other Sunday."

"And still doing so well in school!" her mother said.

This was getting more awkward than regular awkward, so I asked Carly, "How's your school? Connetquot?"

Carly quickened her short gulp of milk, wiping her mouth with a red-and-white napkin with horses on it, and said, "Cliques. Lots of 'em. Little ones and big ones."

"Are you in one of them?" I asked.

"We raised her better than that," her mother answered for her.

"Do you want to meet Zeus?" Carly asked, saving the day as she stood, putting down her glass, and pushing the chair back into the table.

"Sure. I've never met a horse," I said to her mother's obvious pleasure.

"Never met a horse! Well, I think you're in for a treat! He's a good 'un," her mom said, laughing. "You're welcome back here anytime you want, Jerry. It's very nice meeting you. You're as nice as your father."

I gathered up my nice self and my camera and walked out of the house with Carly, the two of us suddenly enveloped for the first time with the feeling of being alone together. We were hyper aware of each other, of the location of our hands, the breathing of our bodies, and the fact that we didn't know much what to say to each other as we walked closer to where Zeus lived. At least that's what I felt and imagined she felt: Our molecules were standing next to each other, regarding each other, and talking, even if the rest of both of us looked quiet.

Zeus's stall was fragrant with a mixture of manure, hay, and earth, which enveloped us as we approached, and he started snorting in anticipation. I hadn't even noticed that Carly had grabbed an apple for him and had it in her right hand, but Zeus noticed it. His nostrils flared, and he pawed at the ground as Carly and I came near, and he held his lips out to her to meet the apple he'd seen.

"Zeus, this is Jerry. Jerry, this is Zeus," she said, gesturing between us, before giving him his midday snack. Zeus's eyes seemed to narrow slightly in pleasure as he gobbled up the apple, big white teeth chomping into it. Carly rubbed his face and his ears, and the sounds of a happy horse crunching an apple filled the stall. There was no place else I'd rather be. There was nothing else I wanted to be doing.

"Good boy," Carly purred. "What a good, good boy."

"Is it okay to take pictures?" I asked.

"Sure. He would like it. Wouldn't you, Zeus? Say cheese!"

"He can just be himself. He's handsome and happy already." I started snapping away. Horse from different angles. Horse with Carly holding the apple. Carly's hand, his mouth. Carly with Zeus in background. Then just Carly.

The door to the stall swung open, and Zeus pulled back in a swirl of reaction. It was Carly's mother. "I'm going to go shopping. Will you two be okay without me? Is there anything you want, Carly, that you didn't put on the list?"

"ChapStick."

"Oh, I can ask Samantha to bring that home from the pharmacy," her mom said, exiting.

"Nothing else."

"Help yourself to whatever is in the fridge. There's lemonade in the pitcher. Sorry to have to run out on you!" she said, waving to me with the tips of her fingers.

It didn't take more than three seconds after we heard the sound of her car pulling out of the driveway before we realized we were alone. *A-lone*.

"Do you want to take Zeus out for a ride?" Carly asked.

I looked at Zeus, and he looked at me. I think I was looking for guidance and direction. He seemed to be telling me something. I took it in, even though I couldn't put it into words right away. They finally came to me. "Maybe we could go inside first, and ride him when it gets a little cooler?"

"Get some lemonade?" she asked.

"Absolutely," I said.

Zeus seemed to nod.

I took three pictures of her as we were walking in, profiles all and one from a few feet in front of her. She shook her head at me saying, "I can't believe you'd want a picture of me in this dirty sweatshirt. I smell like a horse stall."

"It doesn't matter in photography. You can't smell it. Plus it's black-and-white."

When we got inside, we walked right through the kitchen, neither of us stopping for lemonade. She took my left hand and walked me into her room.

"Could you put down the camera?" she asked, laughing, as I quickly snapped two more pics.

She reached over and slipped the camera strap off me, lifting it over my head, then putting my camera on her desk.

Then she took off her sweatshirt. Beneath it she wore a sleeveless V-neck T-shirt of white cotton. I could smell some powdery female scented underarm deodorant – no Right Guard or Old Spice here – mixed with the tang of her sweat. I wasn't sure, but I think beneath her t-shirt was a bra of some sort.

Before I could get that clarified, Carly swept me up in

a fast hug and we leaned, then fell, onto her bed, suddenly all arms and movement, our faces rubbing up against each other, as if we were taking the lead from some other parts of us, waiting for whatever happened next to be broadcast to the top parts of us.

Messages received, after a few more moments of wrestling, this time with our legs entwined, finding their ways into all sorts of nooks and crannies of both of us. We kissed. Better kissing than I'd ever experienced. A different kind of kissing. The not really knowing the person kind of kissing, but finding them out through kissing. I had the strong understanding that if we kept kissing – longer, harder, better – everything else in the world would sort itself out, as this was the first thing that had to happen.

Somewhere in all this, Carly had unbuttoned my shirt; I sat up to take it off and threw it over the chair near her desk. Seeing my camera, I grabbed it and snapped three fast pictures of the delicious, swirling form of her on her bedspread, her arm obscuring her face as she brushed her hair out of the way, then her face, flushed, smiling, and daring.

She turned over on her side and the third picture was of her long frame in those ripped jeans, her t-shirt above it, framed as the living sculpture of desire. I put the camera down and joined her again, in the embrace that had no particular direction other than itself. Now and then we'd come up for air and wrestle around some more. Our breathing had changed, and the air around us seemed different. I wasn't thinking about where this was going. We were already there.

Rolling around, I grabbed my camera again. Without me asking, she seemed to understand that my camera had become part of the moment between us, and she unbuttoned the top of her jeans, sliding them down a whole bunch, so that her sweet panties could be photographed quickly, from the side and the back as she quickly slid over onto her stomach, then she pulled her jeans back up, buttoning them firmly and leaning up toward me, grabbing me by the neck, and embracing me with a strong kiss.

"Maybe we should…"

"What?" I asked nervously, wondering if I'd done something wrong. Or if she wanted more than I'd thought was possible on a school day in daylight.

"Maybe we should ride Zeus to the pharmacy," she said, breaking out into a full smile that made her look older and wiser than we both were.

"Okay. Why not?" I asked.

We got up, and she smoothed over her bedspread. We both smiled and as she turned to put her sweatshirt back on, I caught her in a half-whirl and hugged her tight. She gave me a kiss as if we'd been boyfriend and girlfriend for a year or two. She sniffed her sweatshirt, threw it in her hamper, opened her closet and pulled out a blue-and-white patterned riding shirt. She put it on and looked like a catalog ad for it. She took me by the hand, and we walked out of her room and the house.

Watching her saddle Zeus up, putting all the straps and buckles on him as he seemed to nod consent, almost like a dog watching its owner get the leash for a walk, made me feel that I was part of some exotic adventure that my parents had never scripted for me, so I was all in. "What do I have to do?" I asked.

"I'm going to lead him out," she said. "Then I'll get on him. When I tell you to, put your left foot here and swing your right leg over and come up behind me. Then hold onto me. Put your hands on my hips. There's nothing else to do."

After leading him out and closing up the stable I watched Carly glide up onto him, turning to give me my cue. "C'mon up."

I did, my camera swinging left to right as I rose up, settling in behind her, and in what felt like magic, resting my hands on her hips.

"Hold on like *this*," she said, adjusting my grip to reach further around to her belly, my hands almost meeting at her midsection. "Until you get used to the movement."

Zeus had a gentle, confident walk and didn't seem to mind that there were two of us on top of him instead of just Carly. "How fast does he go?" I asked her.

"Oh he can run, but ... you don't want to see that today. You'd probably fly off of him, right, Zeus?" she asked, patting him. "Horses like Zeus can canter at about fifteen miles per hour and flat out gallop? Around thirty."

"How fast are we going now?" I asked, as we turned left onto Montauk Highway, once there was a break in the cars for us to cross to the far side of the small but busy road.

"About four miles per hour."

"Cool," I said, holding her tightly.

"How does it feel?" she asked, turning her head back toward me, smiling.

"Incredible," I said honestly.

"It gets even better."

"It feels like ... we're back in time. Or suspended in time ... riding the horse to the old apothecary store," I said, laughing.

"We should have different names," Carly said. "I should be Martha."

"Who would I be?"

"Benjamin."

Cars were zooming past us, and Zeus held to a steady, confident walk as the *clip-clop* sound merged with the summer heat and motion of the two of us on the saddle. I snapped a whole bunch of pictures up on the saddle. Benjamin and

Martha were where they wanted to be. We saw that we were getting a lot of looks from people in the cars. It didn't matter, because we were cooler than they were.

The pharmacy came into view. "Where do we park him?" I asked.

"There's a post, actually, on the side street right next door," Carly said.

"You've done this before? You tie him up and he waits?"

"Yes. Where else is he going to go without me? He's my guy!"

Zeus seemed familiar with the arrangement as he maneuvered next to the post. Carly talked me through getting hopping off first, and she followed, in one experienced, fluid movement. Looking at her in boots and jeans, I wondered if I was in love.

"I'm coming in to say hi to my sister," she said. "You have to work today, right?"

I'd actually just about forgotten that. On some level, I assumed I'd continue spending the whole day with Carly.

"I'm just staying a minute."

We walked in, pretty sure not to hold hands, but we stood pretty close to each other as we walked in the door and up aisle seven toward the cash register. Samantha was at the cash register and was beaming a big smile when she saw us.

"Hi, you two! How's it going, sis? Zeus out there?"

"Yup. Around the corner. Want us to bring him in?" Carly said.

"No, we're good. Where's Mom?"

"Shopping. She asked that you bring home ChapStick."

"What flavor?" Samantha asked.

"Mint. Or cherry, if they have it."

"Done," Samantha said, writing it down. "One of each." She walked out from behind the counter over to aisle two and grabbed them. She came back and handed them to Carly, who put them in her jeans pocket.

My father was behind the second counter, filling a prescription when he looked up and saw me. "Well, hello, Cowboy," he said, before catching a glimpse of Carly. "Hello, young lady. You must be related to my partner-in-crime, Samantha."

"Nice to meet you," Carly said, sticking out her hand to shake it and suddenly looking and sounding young.

"You're the horse wrangler?" my dad asked. I was getting embarrassed by his corniness. "What's your horse's name? Cochise?"

"Zeus."

"Is he ... the guy from the Trojan Horse story?" my father asked.

"Dad, you're confused. He is was the sky and thunder god."

"Actually, the supreme ruler of all the gods," Carly said.

"That's got to be one special horse," my father said, grabbing another prescription to fill from the *in* box. "Samantha, could you come help with this? Premarin, .45 mg., 1 daily at night, sixty tablets."

"The blue ones," she asked, moving next to then past my father, gently touching him with her hands on his hips as she passed by him to look for the drug on the side shelves.

"Jerry, when you're ready, there are two large boxes of feminine hygiene products that have to come up and get stocked. They're wrapped in plastic still, at the bottom of the stairs. Whenever you're ready. They need to get set up."

"Well I guess I'd better go," Carly said, putting her hands in her pockets and shrugging.

I walked over to her to have a moment to say good-bye. I approached her left ear and whispered, "This was amazing."

She smiled a beautiful ear to ear smile and leaned into me with a little hug, whispering back to me, "Totally agree." Then she pushed away and turned to leave, not wanting to face either her sister or my father before leaving.

"You okay?" Samantha called out.

"All good!" said Carly.

"Tell Mom I won't be there for dinner tonight," Samantha said to Carly's back as she left the store.

"Will do!"

And Carly was gone. It was suddenly time to work. But not before my father said, "Well, you two seemed to get along pretty well."

"Do the newer products go in front or in back of what's there with the feminine hygiene stuff?" I asked. "Modess and Tampax, right?"

And that was it. I worked, and I thought of her and at some point during my shift. I also thought of Kendra. Before my father and I left for the day, I took the last roll of film I shot out of my camera, combined it with the rolls I'd already shot, wrote up the film developing envelope to go out and left it in the outbox for pickup. I took, with my dad's permission, a licorice for the road. This day was excellent.

It was after math class on Friday, second period, that Kendra caught up with me. We were walking towards the band room.

"My mother says she saw you on a horse on Montauk Highway yesterday. Did that happen, or is she crazy?"

"I, um ... yes, I was trying out a horse. I mean, horseback riding."

"I didn't know you were interested in horseback riding. Since when?"

"My parents thought I should try it out," I quickly lied. "They thought I was getting too wrapped up in books."

Kendra laughed sharply. "Um, no offense, but… I don't think you're getting wrapped up in too many books. I might be ... Dave Levin might be, but if anything, you're getting wrapped up in music."

"Good point," I said, content to leave it at that and walk together in the confusing friendship connection we'd had for years, padding on down the hall.

"She said there was a girl in front, on the horse."

"Yup. Might've been. I mean … there was."

"How…?"

"Zeus," I said. "That's the horse. Lives near Connetquot."

"The girl. Who is the girl?"

"I think her name was ... Carly."

"You're not sure? From yesterday? Are you blushing?"

"No, I'm not! I'm genuinely trying to remember. Yes, that was Carly."

"Was she like one of many girls they give you at a stable when you go to sign up for a horse? My mother said, 'I saw Jerry with this very attractive girl on a horse on Montauk Highway yesterday around 4 p.m.' Did you request a very attractive one? Girl! Not horse." Kendra seemed to be enjoying this now.

"Kendra, she's the kid sister of this girl who works at my father's pharmacy, and they all thought I should go on a horseback ride with her because she is some sort of horse expert, and I need to get out of myself. That's what they told me, 'You need to get out of yourself.' So they set up this ride, I went, and … that was that."

"Did you like it?"

"What do you mean?" I now *was* blushing.

"Horseback riding. What did you think I mean?" Kendra bore into me with her eyes, searching. She was still smiling.

"It was fine. I'm not going to go out and buy a horse."

"Are you going to go out and buy a girl? A Carly girl?" The question hung in the air as Kendra spun away to walk down the hall toward her Advanced Placement English class. (Having opted out of that class, I had band.) "Do me a favor?" Kendra asked, turning to look behind her as she walked briskly now. "Don't call. And I don't want any of those little cute notes from you either. See you later, Cowboy."

I felt really bad. It went quickly from feeling badly about Kendra having to hear about it from her mother to feeling badly about myself to wondering what the hell I was supposed to do now with Carly, as I'd been planning on going home and calling her at some point before or after Kendra to thank her for yesterday.

And maybe even to relive some of it over the phone. But now it was clear that that'd be wrong. Or right in a direction that I hadn't been able to consider seriously and still didn't, because if I did, then why did Kendra's feelings matter so much to me? I couldn't get the memory of wrestling with Carly on her bed out of my mind, though, and particularly the heat of the moment in which she unbuttoned her jeans and posed for me, before grabbing me further. It wasn't in my mind. It was in my body.

"Your room is a mess," my mother said when I came home.

"I'm going to clean it this weekend."

"Do you expect me to?" she asked, her eyes narrowing.

"No. Never. Never in a million years would I expect you to do something as demeaning and stereotypically feminine as that, Mom. That would giving in to The Man and enabling another hundred years of oppression, wouldn't it? I think we'll have to wait for me to clean it up."

"When you try to mock and belittle the Women's Movement you do know, I hope, that it ends up only making you look smaller. The Old Boys' Club days are numbered, Jerry. It's up to you to be on the wrong side of history or not."

"It's just a messy room, Mom," I exploded.

"Harriet. Call me Harriet from now on. Obviously you don't respect me as a mom anyway, so... consider me the mother bird who has pushed the baby birds out of the nest. They can learn to fly or get smashed on the rocks. My job is over."

"Thank you, Mom. That seems like a long way from the Jonathan Livingston Seagull stuff. Have you told Jody yet? About the rocks? Or should I?"

"Your father is not who you think he is. He is not a good man. He's not faithful."

"Then why did you marry him?"

"We were kids. Kids do dumb things. You grow up."

"And learn to push little birds out of nests?"

"You wipe the dew out of your eyes and realize you've been had. But there's still time left. But first you have to survive. He's trying to annihilate me. I've hid it from you and Jody, but I can't anymore."

"Are you getting divorced?"

"Yes. But his lawyer won't cooperate. They won't complete the required documents."

"About what?"

"Money."

"Are we going to be poor, Mom?"

"This is not what I wanted to talk about. But I can't keep it from the two of you anymore. My survival is at stake."

"I want to hear Dad's side of this story," I said coldly, leaving to go upstairs. "So far, I don't believe any of it."

I went upstairs and actually resisted slamming the door. I closed it quietly. I took out the two rolls of special reflective black-light glowing tape and spelled out in big letters over my bed: Soft Asylum. It was from The Doors' album "The Soft Parade," in which Jim Morrison sang a plea to find him exactly that: Soft Asylum. I set up the black light and before I turned it on, I lit the burnt-orange smelling copper-colored scented candle next to my bed. I finally angled the blacklight the right way and turned it on.

The result was awesome. I had my safety. I put on The Doors album, listened to the whole thing and didn't come down for dinner. My mother didn't look for me. I didn't hear my father come home til after 12:30 that night.

That Sunday was one in which my father and I would work together. But instead of talking with him about anything, I found myself being comforted by his presence, by us being guys together, getting ready to go off to work, to open up the pharmacy at 10 a.m. on a Sunday, by assembling the Sunday paper sections together the way we did, by coming home together.

There was no Samantha there on Sunday, there was no Alan, and there were no discussions about anything more than licorice, football, and the best system for making change when a customer buys something for $9.32 and gives you a twenty-dollar bill.

But that next Tuesday, I got off the bus to come in to work and immediately saw my father and his partner, Victor, huddled and bent over slightly behind the second prescription counter. They were clearly handling and shuffling something that didn't look like a prescription.

"Where's Samantha?" I asked, trying to get my bearings.

"She went home early," Victor said, sounding fake neutral. "She wasn't feeling well."

"Looks like you and Carly hit it off pretty well," my father said, looking up with a smile – my pictures of Zeus, Carly, and even more of Carly in his hands. He leaned to the right, raising his hands to show Victor the one he was holding, both of them giving knowing glances and nods.

"No complaints there, huh?" asked Victor.

I watched them flip through each of the pictures, quickly skipping over all the ones of Zeus, the ones where he looked happy, knowledgeable, proud, and connected. They paused over the Carly pictures.

"Good-looking girl," my father said.

"She's sixteen," I said. Those were the first words out of my mouth.

"Didn't seem to slow you down," my father said. "I'm not judging. I'm just saying. So is Kendra. Kendra is good-looking, too."

"Have any pictures of her?" Victor asked, chortling.

I walked over to face them. "Could I have my pictures, please?"

"Sure," my father said, gathering them up to put back in the returned film envelope that should've been opened by me, not them.

"How much do I owe you for them? For the developing?"

My father looked confused.

"Dad, maybe you should ask Victor? Come up with a number?" I grabbed the envelope, turned, and walked over to the candy counter. "Oh yeah, and a few of these," I said, grabbing the remaining eight black licorice packages in the box that held ten."That ought to be it for now." I didn't work that day. Or any more days there. I walked out without any further word.

I walked a mile-and-a-half to a far-flung bus stop and sat on the bench, waiting for the westbound bus on Montauk Highway, which would zoom me right past Carly's and Zeus's house, right home, the Soft Asylum. Sitting on the bench, I finally opened the pictures.

A few were blurry, but most of them were excellent. Try as I did, though, I couldn't feel much beyond admiring the composition of the photos and their exposure. Both Carly and Zeus looked great. It looked like an amazing day had happened. An amazing few moments on a walk, in a stable, on a bed, on a horse. I could imagine them being special and full of feeling to someone who was there.

In that moment, I decided that everything my mother had been saying about my father must've been right. I would work on that assumption from then on.

It didn't make me any better able to stand being around my mother, for the remainder of time before college, though. I watched as she reported going through six different lawyers in the divorce, denouncing each one to me, in turn for being part of the Old Boys' Network because they were in league with my father's lawyer.

"How do you know that?" I would ask.

"Because they met together and were talking," she'd say.

"Isn't that what lawyers do? They're doing what they're supposed to do," I explained.

"If you can't see what is going on here, Jerry, then you are just another part of it. I'm sorry to say it; I had hoped for more from you. But not expected it."

I called Carly to thank her for our time. We both sounded removed from the situation. She didn't ask about the pictures, and though we said we'd get together sometime soon, we never did.

But as I sat in the Soft Asylum many weeks and months later, music filling my increasingly lonely head, heart, and body, I could remember and see Zeus, the horse, supreme ruler of all gods. He had looked at me, into me, and nodded.

Natural Causes

# #

I returned to piano lessons with Mrs. Ketcham on a limited basis, because I accepted that there might be a link between the music I was playing in my band and some of the things she'd been teaching me and making me practice. But I wasn't going to do it the old way. We'd see each other once a month – that was it. That was all she was going to get from me, and that was all I was getting to get from her. Mrs. Ketcham seemed to accept that; at least she got to see me and see that my piano technique wasn't evaporating, even if it wasn't accelerating anymore.

She seemed to switch me towards gentler music, such as Debussy, just as Primeval Ooze was getting into Jimi Hendrix and Black Sabbath. Debussy had no edges, no thunder; he was soft, and everything flowed with ease. I found myself not really wanting or able to play him. Mrs. Ketcham seemed to want the part of me that had gone away. Maybe it was a part neither of us had really seen.

She pulled back and retrenched, trying to train me once again to play the most precious creations of her passionate lover from afar, Beethoven. Maybe the link between Beethoven and Hendrix was closer than the link between my fingers and my heart.

Primeval Ooze was playing more than Catholic Youth Organizations now. We were at private house parties, events at colleges, beach clubs, and country clubs. I think I was the first Jew to step foot into Oceans Ahoy! Country club in Bay

Shore, and public school dances. It was at one of these school dances that I first noticed Deanna.

She wasn't one of the enthusiastic, bouncy, hair swirling while dancing types. She was a weirdo. It looked like she was evaluating our music and our selves, rather than dancing, or deciding to get caught up in it. I later learned this was sheer awkwardness on her part. She was terrified at social events, so decided to act superior to every else around her.

Deanna lived in fear that someone would start up a conversation with her and that she'd be asked to respond in human language. Her dark hair came down on both sides of her face to her shoulders. Her eyes were shielded behind large glasses. Her beauty – and there was beauty – reminded me of all the movies when the guy took off the girl's glasses, brushed her hair back, and said, "My God, Debbie, you're beautiful! How did I not see it?"

So Deanna stood in the corner at the East Islip High School dance staring at me, and I sat behind the Farfisa, my speaker swirling with the solo to "Evil Ways," and we somehow connected without saying anything. At the end of the night, she walked over and stood nearby as I was packing up.

"Hey," I said.

"Hey."

That was about it. She might've said something else before I asked if she went to East Islip High School. This was a pretty dumb question, because we were playing at East Islip High School and everyone at the dance was from East Islip High School.

"Yes. But I didn't have to pay to get in," she said, "I told them I was with the band. I walked in right behind you."

This got my attention, but not too much. Deanna seemed intent on being kind of flat-out wacko. In the right mood, it might strike me as wacko in an attractive way, but right then, she struck me as wacko in an annoying way.

"See you around," I said, happy to be getting on home and counting out my pay from the night. (We were up to about $35 a guy now that we'd made the big time.) I went home and almost forgot about her.

The first long letter from her came at school in science class. It didn't cross my mind that a girl my age would write a really long letter to me. Ever. Deanna had sent it in a sealed envelope put into a larger envelope to her friend Susan, who was in my science class. The letter was all about how hard it was for her to have moved to New York from Indiana, how unfriendly people were, and how constantly annoying her mother and father were with their religious ways in her family, how bleak the world was, and how no one wanted to make it better. I wrote back nicely and said it must be hard to make such a move cross-country.

The next morning, my mother made an unexpected entrance to the kitchen while I was getting ready for school, interrupting me as I was reading the newspaper while eating frozen Reese's Peanut Butter Cups for breakfast. I had gotten used to taking care of myself on school mornings, and I liked the quiet. *Just another perk of feminism*, I thought.

She left me alone. No mom breakfasts anymore. The *New York Times* was reporting on The Pentagon Papers and what they were calling the secret news behind the war in Vietnam.

"Your father is moving out."

"Again?" I asked, staring at her.

"This time for real. It's permanent."

The few months he had returned to the house, following their trial separation, hardly had registered on me. When my father had come home, their separation having ended, he was never home. Thursday nights were the North Patchogue

Fire Department Band, Friday nights were the poker games with Al Spisato and the guys, Wednesdays were The Stock Club (they'd make believe buying and selling stocks, getting make-believe rich, I guessed), he worked til 9:30 p.m. Tuesday nights, and Monday nights depended on the schedule of the other pharmacist, who often seemed to want time off to spend with his family. I don't remember seeing him home on Saturdays and he worked Sundays nine-a.m. to two p.m. The difference between him being home and moving out seemed invisible to me.

"Where is he going?"I asked

"You'll have to ask him that question," my mother said, turning away from me. "By the way: You missed putting the garbage out. We don't ask you for much, could you please do it?" she asked before leaving.

 I didn't verify my mother's report with my father, but the next Saturday, my father said he needed help carrying his belongings out of the house to his car. He didn't have enough suitcases, so what wouldn't fit in them, he'd stuffed into Pathmark shopping bags. He and I went upstairs and downstairs three times, bringing the bags to his '68 GTO convertible. We didn't say anything, just tried hard to make sure the bags didn't rip. The GTO was a cool, aquamarine-colored car with a roaring engine. The thing throbbed in your driveway when you turned the key. He had let me drive it several times in my junior year of high school and told me it'd be mine someday.

I did my best to show him I could drive it well and wasn't some wild, irresponsible long-haired kid with a crazy amount of horsepower under his foot. Still, I loved to drive it around town, blasting some old Beatles song, like "Day Tripper."

We stood in front of the car in silence. I don't know if I was imagining it, but it looked as if my father had a lot to say but couldn't figure out how to do that, so instead, he'd remain quiet. That was the way he usually was. I knew he was happy when he was playing his saxophone, and I could hear his feelings when he played songs like "Misty" or "Nature Boy," but I couldn't figure out what was going on inside him the other times. And the other times were about 95 percent of his life nowadays.

Then he got tearful for a moment. He found his way with words. "I'm not going to be far away, you know, and you're always welcome to come see me. It's not like, y'know..." Then the words stopped, and his eyes swelled with tears for a half-second before he went back to being the guy who seemed to have more to say than he could. Maybe he would someday.

I nodded my head deeply to reassure him that I wasn't secretly aligned with my mother over whatever had happened between them. I told him that I, too, wouldn't be far away, and he was always welcome to see me.

I didn't think we were supposed to hug, so we stood around instead. We both had decided to make this not some big emotional moment. Things would go on, only instead of him not being home almost all of the time, he'd be not home all of the time.

"So... do you work this Sunday?" I asked.

"Yes. Nine to two, the usual. You always know you can get me at the pharmacy."

Then he walked toward me for some kind of hug, and we held onto each other awkwardly. I could feel his chest give a single heave. Then he patted me three times on the back, and he pulled away.

He got in the car, whose top was down, the Pathmark bags in the back seat making it look like some sort of festive summer outing for old clothes and shoes was at hand. He turned the key, the engine throbbed, and he drove off.

It took me a while to realize that he hadn't said where he'd be living.

Almost as soon as he moved out, our household was brittle and felt angry. My mother was at odds with my sister a lot, arguing about everything from whether or not Jody was allowed to hang around the roller skate rink ("You just hate it because there are black and Puerto Rican people there! Admit it!") to morning arguments about clothing, the clothes dryer, homework, etc. ("Why didn't you wash the pants that *don't* make me look fat?" my sister screamed.

"Don't talk to me like I'm one of your friends!" my mother yelled back.)

I kept listening to a lot of music at loud volume that year with my door kept closed. Sometimes in the far background, I could hear my mother and sister arguing.

My mother would play her own music through the downstairs stereo, namely Helen Reddy's "I Am Woman" over and over again. I would walk from my bedroom to the bathroom to brush my teeth and hear Helen Reddy blaring that she was a woman, could do anything, and something about if I didn't want to be on her side, supporting her as a brother supports a sister, get out of the way, because she could roar. *Good morning*, I'd think.

One morning my mother started with me for one reason or another, blasting me for my attitude, which apparently wasn't to her liking since my father left. "Are you familiar with how patriarchy is handed down? Because you are certainly acting like you think you're the *man* of the house," she said accusingly.

"Mom, do you see any others here? Men?" I shot back. "I'm it, right? The lucky winner?"

I had to get out of this place. Short of getting arrested for something and sent away, my best hope was to find something my parents thought would be seen as character-building or a résumé item for college when I applied. I was too old now, to return to Camp Encore (the summer camp in Maine for musical boys), so I looked in the back of newspapers and magazines for bicycling or hiking tours for people my age. It didn't matter where. Anywhere off Long Island.

I found a bike tour in New England. We'd meet up in Boston at Tufts University, and go north from there. There'd be about fourteen of us, along with two guides in their young twenties. The rest of us were sixteen and seventeen. I sent away for the brochures, showed them to my parents in separate meetings (my dad at the pharmacy, my mom in our almost men-free living room). There was enough guilt between the two of them, I guessed, that they agreed to pay for almost all of it. I had to contribute $300 of my own, which I had from my Primeval Ooze earnings. I would be be gone for fourteen days that summer. My sister would be on her own with these people. Good luck, Jody.

Deanna's second letter was waiting for me in science class again via Susan. It spoke about her theoretical speculation about the universe and the implausibility of God. I didn't write back.

She asked, in her third note, two days later, if she could call me that night. I said yes. She spoke for about forty-five minutes about how hypocritical everyone at East Islip High School was, and how her parents and grandparents were strange people who might be considered crazy by some, but who passed easily for normal in Indiana. Out here on Long Island, she said, her parents hunkered down and avoided everyone. Which put more pressure on her, because they were always home.

May was coming, and it would be prom season. Kendra and I had agreed to go to the Islip High School prom a long time ago (ninth grade?) – as either friends or boyfriend and girlfriend; we weren't sure, and we didn't spend time talking about it, even though we both thought the whole prom idea was silly.

But Deanna didn't seem to think proms were silly; they were proof to her that she was an outsider, was ugly, and would never be asked to go by any boy. And East Islip's prom for some reason would be delayed that year, due to school construction and asbestos removal. The date for the prom would actually be after the seniors' graduation. While I thought that might make it easier for Deanna to have the issue fade away as the school year ended and for me to become invisible to her, it didn't. It made her focus more and more on how she didn't fit in and how she needed someone to help her not lose her mind.

So I asked her to go to her prom with me.

I now had two junior proms to go to with two different girls.

I don't *think* I was thinking of sex at the time I asked Deanna. But I might've been. It was clear to both Kendra and me that sex was not on the agenda between us. Maybe it shouldn't have been on anyone's agenda. But it was the summer before my senior year. In two weeks, I'd be with my bicycling group up in Medford, Massachusetts, setting out on adventures on a new Motobecane bike that I'd convinced my parents to buy me if I paid an extra $100 toward it.

But for now – Saturday, July 3, 1971 – I was in the backseat of a limo with Deanna and another couple. Deanna was dressed up in what was supposed to look nice, but to me, she didn't look like herself at all. She looked like an awkward birthday cake. And I looked like the perfect match for her, a game-show host in a rented tux.

I was sitting next to her thinking about how my instinct

had been right, that proms were stupid. That's when I heard on the limo driver's radio station as the last item in the news recap for the 10:00 hour, "And ... in Paris, France, singer/songwriter Jim Morrison of The Doors is dead at the age of twenty-seven, apparently of natural causes." The moment froze me. I felt everything stop.

It was the end of believing that everything around me was changing in a cool direction. It was the end of me believing that my generation would be magically revolutionary and humane and very, very different than the world my father and mother and their divorce lawyers handed me.

There would be no breaking on through to the other side. There would just be getting older, then dying. Someday the music that I loved would be used to sell Cadillacs on TV. The Doors were dead. The Beatles were over. The '60s were a memory. If Morrison was dead at age twenty-seven, then maybe we would all grow up to die before our ugly thirties. "Natural causes."

The other couple continued talking and laughing. Deanna stared at me. I don't remember the rest of the night. It might've been pretty prom, stupid, but not stupid in a special enough way to remember.

Both Deanna and I seemed to feel let down in each other in the weeks that followed. I only got one more letter from her about existentialism, and I didn't understand a word of it. I didn't care. Was *that* existentialism?

I wanted to get my new bicycle and ride it. In my mind I wanted after our New England trip, to keep riding it all the way to Montreal. They had high schools and rock bands up there, too.

I could be Canadian.

The Peach

#

They dug a hole in the ground in late March and set the foundation in April. By May the new red-and-yellow building with big parking spaces and outdoor tables was only about 175 yards away from our high school. The new McDonald's was open for business by the beginning of our junior year with a sign under the yellow arches that blared "Over Seven Billion Sold." And though it was a mere two-minute walk around a duck pond to get to those arches from the school, we weren't allowed to go. Oh, you could go there on a weekend, but not for lunch on a school day.

For that you got to stay in the cafeteria and have mystery meat with vegetable medley, a mealy apple, and a "variety of chilled milks." If you were lucky, you'd watch Joey Zelko either get thrown out for something he'd said or thrown at another kid, or get called down to the office to answer for something he'd thrown or said yesterday.

As Mr. Tuffin, our principal, explained to me calmly, the school, you see, was acting "in loco parentis." He was, I think, hoping that his use of something that sounded Latin and legal would shut me up and make me go away, as I'd become a mouthy student council vice president and advocate for whatever seemed to most annoy him. His secretaries greeted me each time I came down to talk with him with an eye roll, followed by a narrowing of the eyes, and a sharp, "What are you here for? What do you want to see him about?," before telling me that he wasn't available.

Tuffin was supposed to be having meetings with me, monthly, as part of a big overture he made to the student council. After he said his "door was always open" in the first five minutes of his greeting to us, Mercy Belcheck asked if that meant he'd have monthly meetings with us to hear our concerns. Caught off-guard, he'd said, "Sure." Then it turned out no one except me wanted to meet with the guy.

"Why can't we go to McDonald's, if we bring in a note from our parents? Wouldn't that make you non-loco parentis?" I asked. This was clearly the tenth or twelfth annoying thing for him to hear by 8 a.m. this fine October morning, because his face flushed, and he seemed to go quickly from calm to almost choking on anger.

"You can't run a school without accountability. If everyone is walking everywhere they want to go on a given day, then we wouldn't know where anyone was. It defeats the idea of academic periods one through nine and leaves us liable."

I looked at him carefully. He looked almost square. Not like they used the word in the '60s, but literally, physically square, as if one of those old black-and-white photos of administrators in 1951 came to life. "That makes no sense," I argued. "You could still have classes and attendance."

"We *will* have classes. And no one leaves them without permission. If you get hit by a car or kidnapped, or you are a senior and are driving and have an accident, who is responsible?"

"Whoever was responsible for it."

"Wrong answer. We are," he said, looking satisfied.

"The McDonald's is a couple of hundred yards away from the attendance office. How are you going to get kidnapped?"

"You don't think there are bad people out there?"

"Not as many as you do."

"You're willing to have me take that chance?"

"Absolutely."

"Well, the answer is 'no.' When things go wrong, I'm the one that has to answer for it. Not you."

"You know things were different at the Summerhill School. There's a book about it. Education without fear or coercion."

"Where did you hear about this?"

"Psychology class."

He looked annoyed. "I'm glad you are so up-to-date in your actual class curriculum that you have the time to read extra things outside of it," he said. "Where was this school – Sweden?"

"England. They had weekly meetings with the teachers and the students and each person got one vote about how the place would run." My mother had also told me about the place.

"That's ridiculous," Mr. Tuffin snorted. "When was that, the '60s?"

"The 1920s. They wanted to see what happened if they believed in people's goodness," I said.

"Chaos. That's what happens," he said, cutting it short.

"They called it democracy," I said. "I thought that was in the official advertising for this country."

"This country has done pretty well the way we've done it, and we're not going to have chaos at Islip High School, however much you might enjoy that."

Tuffin had been looking for a way to show he was the one and only person truly in charge of our daily existence since we entered the school. He knew that I walked around with the phone number for the American Civil Liberties Union's office in Queens in my pocket ever since he'd told us that any visible signs of protest, in the forms of armbands or political T-shirts wouldn't be tolerated if they expressed dissatisfaction with the Vietnam War or Nixon.

"You're welcome to think whatever you want to think about the war in Vietnam," he'd told me the month before. "You're just not allowed to disrupt others' right to learn."

"Wearing an armband or T-shirt doesn't disrupt anyone's right to learn. Plus ... learn *what*, anyway?" I asked. "Are we going to start learning about Vietnam, true things about it, or are we going to stay with 'Europe and the World Marketplace' forever?"

"You can't wear armbands or make a scene."

"We're not going to make a scene."

"You'll get the football players riled up. Coach Melnick and Cuticelli are ex-marines."

"Good for them. Why aren't they in Vietnam then, if they believe in it?"

"Being a good citizen means respecting others' military service."

"My uncle died fighting in World War Two," I said. "I don't think he would have gone to Vietnam."

"To each his own," he said, looking vaguely disgusted and away from me. "There's not going to be any demonstrations on so-called Moratorium Day."

"You know, the ACLU is looking for new test cases. You could put Islip on the map if you try to impose your pro-war beliefs on the rest of us or stifle our legal expressions in any way."

He took a minute to formulate what he would say to me, fuming, then said, "This isn't Queens. And you aren't going to threaten me or any of us. We've been here a long time, and we will be after you leave. Are we done?"

"Kids have been making suggestions in the student council suggestion box and they want to know why they can't get up to get a drink of water or go to the bathroom without a teacher's permission," I informed him. I wasn't going to let go of a good line of aggravation, hoping he'd just give in on something.

"That's ridiculous," he sputtered.

"I'm talking about going to the water fountain or the bathroom, not McDonald's. I know you think McDonald's is ridiculous."

"There are nine water fountains. There are twelve hundred kids at this school. That's..." he took out an old calculator and punched in the numbers, "over one hundred and fifty-five kids at each water fountain."

"They don't all want water at the same time! They're not all going to walk out at the same time,"

"But they could. They *could*. That's my point. That's the situation you could be looking at. What class do you have now? Who let you out to come here?"

"Study hall and it was Steadman."

"That's it for today; go back to class. Have the secretaries write you a pass."

"There's something else. You said you'd get back to me about the request to have a guest speaker come into social studies class about Angola and Portugal. It's the last European colony in Africa, and they're fighting for their independence. The guy I saw speak said they were like our George Washington, and he's willing to come in and talk."

"He's not coming here to talk. He's not invited."

"Why not?"

"Because he's not George Washington. He's a political figure, and it is one-sided."

"I contacted the Portuguese ambassador's office to the UN, and they said they'd consider sending someone to represent the other side."

"Absolutely not."

"Don't you want two sides represented?"

"I don't want any side represented. I want you to learn the curriculum they are teaching. If the teacher – who is the teacher?"

"Mr. Monita."

"If Mr. Monita wants to supplement it with someone who will come in to talk about African art, or dance or tribal customs, that is something else."

"Will you consider what you just said? Tribal dances and things?"

"I didn't say 'tribal dances.' You are quoting me out of context and mixing it up. You do this every time I speak with you."

"How do you know that?"

"Because I hear what you say about it afterward."

"So you are spying on us?"

"Go back to class *now*. Get a pass."

Angola was my pet project, after I'd heard a speaker at a weekend conference for students about politics and Africa at St. John's University. I should've remembered that no one in Islip cared about Angola. There were only two actual issues the student council wanted me to take up with him, based on the council meetings and little pieces of paper left in the suggestion box near the stairway: They wanted a smoking lounge for seniors (there wasn't a snowball's chance in hell in getting that), and they wanted to be allowed to leave for lunch to go to McDonald's.

No one believed the school cared about us getting kidnapped on the way around the duck pond, or getting in car accidents at 11:52 in the morning. What we all believed – what we all knew – was that the administrators were afraid that kids were going to go out for lunch, get high or do drugs, *then* have hamburgers and milkshakes and hot apple pies. Kids either would come back into the building useless, giggling stoners or violently assaultive LSD-munching rebels, or ... just not come back at all. So in preparation for the worst possibility – that they'd be forced to let us out for lunch – Tuffin brought in some heavy backup.

The two Frankensteins appeared in the hallway late October. They were Suffolk County cops – well, retired cops. They walked stiffly, oddly stuffed into suits and ties, their long cufflinked arms not at ease by their sides. They had really short hair, the kind absolutely no one outside of the military wore. They snooped around and learned the intersections, the previously hidden hallway nooks where students gathered to make out or hand things to each other. Their gaze gave away nothing, other than they would use force against you if they had to, and that it wouldn't disturb their day in the least if they had to. It might even improve it.

Our school was the first in the county to hire cops instead of nice old ladies or retired woodshop teachers to do the patrolling. The word was that they were drinking buddies of Mr. Melnick, who had brought in a young marine who was home on leave to tell our class that we were winning the war in Vietnam and that it would be over in a few months anyway, because we were looking at the light at the end of the tunnel now.

That was five years ago, in sixth grade. The war was not only still going on, it was escalating and it looked to me that we were losing it while killing lots of civilians. *Life* Magazine had double-page color pictures of dead mothers, babies, and older children laying on the side of the road. They'd been killed fleeing their homes by the U.S. Army. Between 200 and 500 of them in an hour. None of them had weapons.

We all knew we had to register for the draft when we

turned eighteen, because they needed new people to send to Vietnam every year. I knew I wouldn't be going anywhere to shoot unarmed people. But I might be going to college in Montreal. I would miss New York bagels, pizza, and the beach.

Jimmy Hoffa's Teamsters union and the construction workers made a big show of appearing at antiwar rallies in cities in hard hats with baseball bats, starting fights or beating anyone who had long hair and was against the war. They screamed at them to get haircuts, take a shower, get a job, or to go to Russia, and see how they liked it there.

"Love it or leave it" meant accepting the war and agreeing to kill whoever old men told you to kill. Rabbi Dobin in Bay Shore had developed a reputation for writing letters certifying kids as conscientious objectors when it came time for Vietnam. But you had to convince him that you were opposed to using violence in general – in all wars. I knew this wasn't true for me. I would've fought in Europe or against Japan twenty-five years ago, as my uncle had.

The few of us who took the time to learn about the war pretty much knew how Mr. Melnick and Coach Cuticelli's football team felt about the war. But we really found out when seven of us wore black armbands to school protesting the war, on Moratorium Day, joining with a nationwide swell of protests at high schools and colleges.

"Hey, faggot! You scared of going to Vietnam? You scared of fighting gooks, you commie? You like gooks more than your own people?" Football players always traveled in pairs or threesomes, so they didn't have to feel personally responsible when they spit on you.

Then, not three weeks later, we learned that the former high school quarterback of the varsity team had been killed in action. No one said anything about it.

"The Frankensteins are here for drugs," Greg Lefliger said. "They think it's the juniors and seniors. They can smell weed a half-mile away."

"Like they're upright drug-sniffing dogs?" I asked.

"Not as nice. These guys will plant stuff in your locker if they don't like you," he said, nodding slowly. "Dogs just want a Milk-Bone."

"Or weed."

"Yeah, but they get a Milk-Bone if they find weed."

Tuffin always seemed personally offended by the existence of long hair, free speech, girls in short skirts, guys in shorts, weed, and any faculty members who weren't in their fifties.

Gary, my old friend from the days of camping out on his side lawn, looking at *Playboy* days, had moved on to reading Timothy Leary and dropping acid. We walked the shortcut home from school on a Friday in September, neither of us intending to do any optional reading assignments for homework this weekend. "Screw that. You've got to read *The Politics of Ecstasy*, man," he said, nodding. "Timothy Leary."

"Why?"

"It's like an acid trip, but in print."

"I don't want to do acid," I said, remembering I'd seen something about some girl throwing herself off of a rooftop because someone told her she could fly while on LSD.

"You've read all those stories about bad trips?" he asked. "They're all made up. They are fake. It's Nixon law-and-order bullshit."

"Art Linklater's daughter?"

"Yeah, she killed herself, but they did an autopsy, and there weren't any drugs in her system."

"I'm not doing acid, Gary."

"Fine. So you're going to drink Boone's Farm Apple

Wine or Mateus and get enlightened or something? You're just going to get drunk."

"What do you mean 'enlightened'?"

"When you are on acid, Leary points out, and you are holding a peach, you just ... really know it is a peach."

"I already know that, Gary."

"No you don't. You think you do. Trust me."

"What does any of this have to do with stopping the Vietnam War? Or social justice, ending racism, those things? How is that going to happen? Are you going to just tell them about the peach?" I asked.

"You don't tell anyone anything. They experience it. It has to do with the cortex," he said, pointing to his head. "You know the Hendrix album? *Are You Experienced*? What do you think he is talking about?"

"I thought it was about sex," I half-lied.

"Yeah, well, it isn't. Think about it," Gary said, before walking away in the direction of his house, the last time I ever saw him. "And listen to the song. Listen better."

"Will do," I said.

I went home and said hello to my mother. "Tonight is garbage night," she said.

"Uh-huh," I said, before heading upstairs to my records.

I found the track "Are You Experienced"; it was weird to have a song as a question. Four minutes and thirteen seconds. Backward sounds. A pounding guitar. Encouragement to get my mind together, an invitation to hold hands, and watch the sunrise from the bottom of the sea. One note pounding on a piano somewhere in the background. A voice asking if I'd ever been experienced... if I'd ever been beautiful.

I said good-night to my my mother a few hours later, hours that were kind of lost in time as I started flipping through two books I'd bought because Deb Vanettle said I should know them, and they were woven into existentialism, even if they weren't actually existentialist: *Steppenwolf* and *Narcissus & Goldmund.*

I read them. Strange names abounded, but I got that these were, underneath it all, people like me, and my parents, and Gary, and that the world they were in wasn't mine, but wasn't fixed in time either, as anything that truly separated us because the things that I thought were fixed in time and my life – -things like Ethan Allen furniture, bar mitzvahs, high school dances, and painted polka dots on the walls on the way downstairs to our finished basement (my mother's latest home based creative art project) weren't any more real than hallucinatory excursions into another realm, this one with a Long Island address. Maybe Gary had a point and a peach *was* a peach, across centuries and continents.

Things were hidden and things were also obviously, exactly what they seemed.

I put on The Doors' album and listened to "Soul Kitchen," and when it got to the invitation to sleep all night in someone's soul kitchen, I got choked up. I needed that, someone, somewhere warmer and bigger, than my quietly disintegrating family, my stupidly controlling school, the military fighting force that would want me. The song was calling, and coaxing me, telling me to learn how to forget. How do you do that? Learn to forget?

Of all the things I wanted to forget, being a nice guy was top of the list. I'd already had a few girls tell me how nice I was, while they focused their attention on dangerous dirtbag kids in our same grade. All that being nice got me seemed to be a pat on the head from teachers and a reminder to throw out the garbage on Wednesday nights.

The not-so-nice guys, who were just a little older than

I was, were getting drunk, high, feeling up girls, joining in college demonstrations against the war, going to Steppenwolf concerts, throwing their fists in the air, singing "Born to Be Wild"... I was listening to Kendra play the new Joni Mitchell album for me and respectfully keeping my hands to myself, even when she came home in an Islip Buccaneers' cheerleader outfit one day.

(I literally couldn't figure out what she was wearing under that short, pleated skirt, and I didn't do anything to find out. I figured that's what you were supposed to do as a nice guy. Look, but don't touch. Or maybe as a nice guy I wasn't even supposed to be thinking this way. I wasn't even an *effective* nice guy.)

A nice guy was also supposed to follow Tuffin's directives and allow my high school to groom us for Vietnam and kill people who like Narcissus and Goldmund lived in their different world but who, underneath it all, had families and dreams just like us. Thousands and thousands of them were and would be killed by people like the kids in my community, a few years older than us, now, this year, and the next.

And I'd come to understand that it wasn't enough to be quiet and nice about the war. People needed to be disrupted before they would consider new thoughts, new ways. And that's when I started planning the walkout. We'd do it late in the day – ninth period – but we'd walk out of classes, walk out of the school, and not even go to McDonald's. We'd go to the town park, walk down Main Street with signs, walk past Louie's' Luncheonette, past the pharmacy, past the bank, and we'd assemble on the square. What could they do, arrest us?

But first was the issue of "us." There wasn't really an "us." It was me. And a few kids I knew from the lunchroom. About six of them.

I thought lots of kids might want the chance to raise their

voices, through action, to show their opposition to the war. I was pretty sure they'd also want to walk out of school with a bunch of other people and some of them would head straight to McDonald's.

I went into school the next morning after downing my usual frozen mini-Reese's Peanut Butter Cups and orange juice for breakfast and looked for Gary, to tell him about my Narcissus and Goldmund thoughts, but he wasn't there. The two Frankensteins, though, were there, right in front of his locker, emptying it. I hadn't seen anything like that before, so I asked them where he was. The taller one snorted and the other one said, "Get to class."

I was concerned enough to ask the school nurse if she'd seen him or if he was okay, and she directed me to the guidance counselor, Mr. Beck. Mr. Beck had the largest bald head I'd ever seen on a person and always wore a suit and a tie. Every time he talked, he made it sound like he wasn't supposed to be sharing this information with you, but was willing to anyway, so today was no different.

"Gary is going away for a little while," he said, nodding slightly.

"Where to?"

"I'm not at liberty to say."

"Is he all right?"

"Privacy regulations mean that I can't talk about it," he said.

At lunch, it was Roman Lubov who told me: Gary had been busted for selling LSD during French class. He'd been taken away in a squad car after his parents came in. The cops had already cleaned out his locker, after finding fifteen hits of acid in the jacket pockets of his fringe jacket hanging inside. "We ain't gonna see him again," Roman said, laughing.

I gnawed at the tasteless chocolate chip cookie the school

lunch had provided for dessert. Roman slurped down his fruit cup in one fast move.

"You gonna eat that?" he asked, pointing to my other dessert. "That's a fruit cup, right?"

"It's peaches in syrup," I said. "Yeah, I'm gonna have it."

It was dripping in sweetened liquid, but still crunched a bit and looked the right color. That was all I had to go on to identify it as having once been a peach.

"Did you hear about the walkout to McDonald's?" Roman asked. "It's on for period nine."

When the walkout finally happened, there were about seven of us who walked through town holding our signs. McDonald's took the bulk of our walkouts. A good number of kids left school and went wherever.

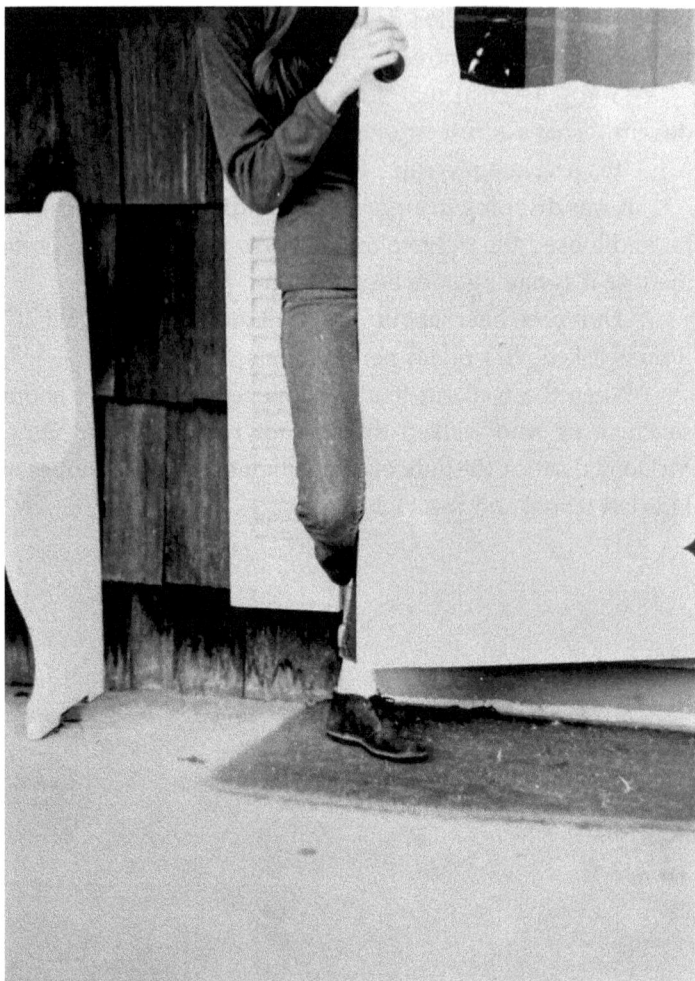

In the Garden

# #

Fleeing Long Island and my parents' divorce-in-progress, I left on a sunny July day to meet my new bike, a burgundy Motobecane. I nicknamed him François because of his obvious French heritage. I'd met him on the lawns of Tufts University, where he was being assembled by the tour group's leaders, Chuck and Davis.

I finally met the other teens whose names I'd had on a list they mailed to me just before the prom with Deanna. Each of these kids had fled his/her own hometowns to gather here in New England. The standouts to me were Lincoln, an aggressive rider from Conway, New Hampshire, who actually had a beard at age seventeen and always wore a headband; Fiona, a twinkly-eyed spiritual sprite from Portland, Oregon, who I would learn loved Maine when it rained – she would try to start a campfires in the rain while the rest of us cursed and complained from our soggy/leaking pup tents; and Sam, a friendly gravel-voiced blond guy from Georgia who could assemble or disassemble a ten-speed bike while sleeping.

I introduced myself to them and our group leaders, and we watched the wrenches whirl as seats got assembled, lights put on, and brakes adjusted. I took François out for a spin around the parking lot and went zipping past some of the empty for summer college halls. I felt powerful; we could do this for *miles*, François and me. We were a long way from Long Island.

Then Lisa arrived.

She was blonde, had a warm Middle American smile, and the longest, most athletic legs I'd seen on anyone our age. I had to consciously tell myself to stop staring as her white shorts showcased the creamy-tan contours of her legs as she waved nervously at us all, laughing and introducing herself as being from Grosse Pointe, Michigan.

I felt sorry for her coming from a place with such a silly name. Much later I found out that her family was wealthy, and she lived in one of the more exclusive neighborhoods in the whole country. I didn't know about many towns outside of Long Island.

Lisa wanted to study art history in college, she said, and wanted senior year to go as quickly as possible. Her parents were *not* divorced, seemed to love each other, and did things like surprise her with sudden news about everyone going to Barbados. She'd already asked them for a trip to Europe after her senior year to see famous artworks in person.

The sunny, rainy, sweaty July into August days of our New England riding tour went quickly. Jefferson had to be sent home, after it was discovered he'd sprayed Off insect repellent onto one of his peanut-butter-and-jelly sandwiches in a creative suicide attempt. François and I spent our days swerving and swaying and zooming through all small towns, the wind in my face, trying to remain in close proximity to Lisa and her athletic pumping legs whenever possible.

The towns were small, and the roads were deliciously smooth with lots of good hills. Every time we'd take any riding breaks at all, Lisa and I seemed to be near each other. We talked about our lives, and it became easier each time. We talked about our parents a whole bunch, her brother, my sister, and how alternately confusing and shallow high school now seemed. College would be different.

I learned on the trip, that I liked Salem, Massachusetts,

a lot, that New Hampshire actually has a beach coast (for thirteen miles anyway), that Maine is awful in a pup tent when it rains for three days in a row, no matter what Fiona said or sang around her half-started weak campfire, and most of all, that Lisa was a magnetic force for me. No calculation or right words were necessary to bring us together. We just attracted. And moved toward each other with it. This felt different. It was happening.

The trip ended, and it was harder for me to say good-bye to Lisa than I expected. We stood in front of each other smiling a lot, then she leaned in to give an almost best-friend hug. We exchanged addresses and phone numbers and vowed to see each other during senior year.

Only after I returned home alone I realized that Lisa was to me the first girl who wasn't Kendra whom I saw as a full, real person you could talk to. And listen to. Talking with Lisa made me feel better about being alive, living in my family, and not having a clue about what to do after graduation. She was in a category of her own, because even though Kendra had the same qualities, unspoken limits had been put in place (for years now) that showed where the guardrails were. No such limits had been discovered or declared with me and Lisa. All things were possible

In every exchange of letters between Lisa and me, the magnetic pull strengthened, and we both knew this meant sexually as well. Sometimes I would hold her letter in my hand, taking in all the textures of her handwriting, return address in Connecticut, choice of stamp, looking at the reverse of the letter, imagining her licking it before sealing it and sending it, and then I would open it and read it, rereading it as soon as I got done, laying back on my bed, then staring at my ceiling, realizing that I really had connected with her and that we would find a way to see each other soon. We would.

I knew we would. We had to find an excuse, a weekend that my mother wouldn't be around, and a way.

The first break came when my mother scheduled a March weekend to go visit her friend, Joan, in New Jersey. I squawked about having to look after Jody, and my mother urged her to go to her friend Caroline's house for those two days "so your brother can be as selfish as he wants without impacting you."

The excuse at Lisa's end was searching for colleges. Even though she had centered her college search on Boston-area schools, she quickly added Hofstra to it. "Safety school," she told her parents. She would drive down carefully and stay overnight with someone from last year's New England bicycling tour.

She told her parents she'd be staying with Stacy, who in fact lived on Long Island, too. Though I'd never really even noticed Stacy on the trip, Lisa and she had enough of a positive connection that Stacy got on the phone with Lisa's mother and assured her that she was perfectly welcome to stay with her that weekend. She said her parents would be home and would be happy to see her with a friend staying over. And that was all it took.

We were both virgins and somehow had talked about that. We both researched birth control, but came up with different solutions. That meant we were bringing slightly different stuff to the event. She brought spermicidal cream and I brought lubricated spermicidal condoms. One thing we had in common was a mission to massively kill sperm wherever they were to appear. We lit the scented candle and turned on the blacklight and chose the right incense, our baby-preventing tools at the ready, and with the help of a few sips of Mateus white, we kissed. And kissed some more. Then we danced around and kissed. Dancing stopped, and we pressed our bodies up against each other. We were still led by our kisses. Once moaning started we were goners: This was going to happen. It *was* happening; today, right here, right now.

I had some quiet feeling that whatever was missing from our lives – from my life as a guy, from the way I thought and felt and moved, to hers as a nice girl from Michigan who loved art, would be found by Lisa and I becoming lovers. The center of her meeting the center of me. A garden would be there for both of us.

And it was. We both took off our shirts. After much nervous laughter and some joking, we took off everything else. Getting under the covers in my bed slowed us down as we got warm all over again and tried to comprehend that we were truly naked with someone of the opposite sex, and not just someone, but someone we liked! A good kisser, for the first time in our lives.

Totally nervous about it being her first time, too, I didn't want to hurt her. We figured that the slower and slippier, we could go, the better our chances of avoiding pain and maximizing pleasure would be. So out came all the slippery stuff. I was so distrustful of all the provisions that I suggested we use *two* condoms at once, just in case, and she agreed.

So there we were, super-lubed up and slick and wrapped tightly (twice over), all ready to go. Somehow we still wanted each other despite all the careful preparations. We resumed kissing each other and were thrilled to touch each other. Suddenly going all the way felt so good and natural and inevitable that it didn't even seem like a different idea or event than the rest of it. Only it was. It was *doing it, The Real Thing,* which added excitement onto the layer of celebrating our kisses and our nakedness and our daring and no one being home but us. We were in a place of our own creation together, a liaison of fun, slippery friction, mounting tension, kisses, heartbeats, and,finally, release. We hugged each other and cried, kissing again.

We had been each other's first time and we were grateful that it was someone as nice and kind and exciting and decent and good-looking and sweet-tasting as each other. After laughing and laying there for a while, we did it again, because we could and wanted to.

We went on to become deep long-distance friends in our senior year and first year of college. We didn't think about going to the same college or altering our individual plans in any way. We wrote letters to each other about the important things in our lives, and how these were changing. There was no talk of marrying each other or devoting our lives to each other. Maybe we'd discovered a charged-particle solar system together, but there was a universe out there for each of us to inhabit.

Silence

# #

I went to the college my father wanted me to attend. It was an Ivy League college; his dream come true. I watched as nine of my eleven friends dropped out, shortly before I did, too. Either it was the wrong place, or I was the wrong person.

When I returned home, I called to ask Mrs. Ketcham if I could visit with her.

"Of course! Without delay," she said.

I no longer had a bike to ride to lean against the tree in the front yard while with her, so I borrowed my mother's car and drove there.

I knocked and Mrs. Ketcham opened the door, holding it open with a big smile on her face. I came in and she hobbled away with her familiar creakiness, leading us to the chairs in front of the old piano we spent so many hours with. She was clearly much stiffer and slower now, aging fast. "Do you still play?" she asked.

"I do."

That felt like the litmus test; I had passed. I felt proud of it.

"What kind of music?" she asked with a look of genuine curiosity on her face that I'd never seen before.

"Can I show you?" I asked.

For the next twenty minutes, I played her abbreviated versions of Ray Charles, Leon Russell, Iron Butterfly, Procol Harum, and Doors songs I'd learned. We sat next to each other, just as when she'd first shown me duets. I finished. It was quiet. I looked at her and could see that she didn't know what to say. It was a sweet type of confusion.

But she was teary. I was, too. I don't know how, but we both knew this would be the last time we saw each other.

"I don't know where you will end up, but I hope you will keep playing. It is a wonderful companion as you age. No one can take it away from you."

It was my turn to not know what to say.

"If your hair were shorter, it would be better," she said, touching my hair, wiping a tear of mine away, and brushing my hair behind my ear. "See?" she said. "I can see your face."